As you encounter Jerrod [...] Chains," you will grow to lo[...] to first meet Jerrod in 2[...] enthusiasm and passion for [...] *seminars and appeared on national television together. He will lead you on the pathway to optimal health as he shares his journey with you.*

Olin Idol, N.D., C.N.C.
Author of Pregnancy, Children and The Hallelujah Diet

Jerrod's story of survival has been an inspiration to many. I admire his passion for educating people to help them make more informed choices to improve their health and the quality of their lives.

Jeff Rogers
Author of Vice Cream

After nearly 15 years beyond a terminal cancer diagnosis, Jerrod continues to be an inspiration on healthy eating and living. He is a true example of mind-body discipline to follow and admire.

Alan Furmanski
Publisher and Writer

Jerrod and Nikki are living examples of how great life can be when we eat to live. It is an honor to know that some of the recipes I created are among their favorites. If you are ready to be inspired for life, then this book is a must read.

Sarma Melngailis
Author, Living Raw Food and Raw Food, Real World
Proprietor, Pure Food & Wine | One Lucky Duck, New York City

When I met Jerrod and Nikki back in 2003 our families spent a delightful afternoon together. Since then we have remained in contact and periodically gotten together. What Jerrod most reminds me of is "hope." He has always struck me as a "find-a-way" kind of guy. And he's always trying to pass along the hope that he has to others. Too many of us give up our dreams and settle for a lot less than God envisioned for us. Let Jerrod inspire you, instruct you, and make your hope come alive again.

Michael Donaldson
Director of Research, Hallelujah Acres

FOODCHAINS.INFO

JERROD SESSLER

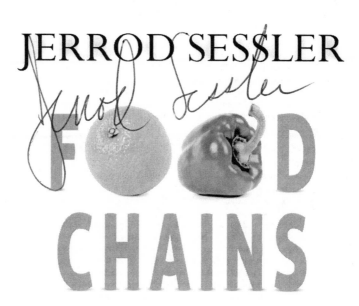

FOOD
CHAINS

Break Free & Enjoy Life

ToDoBlue
PRESS

SEATTLE, WASHINGTON

Food Chains by Jerrod Sessler

First Edition

Copyright © 2013 by Jerrod Sessler

All rights reserved. Except as permitted under the U.S. Copyright Act of 1976, no part of this publication or associated work by the author or publisher may be reproduced, distributed, or transmitted in any form or by any means, or stored in a database or retrieval system, without the prior written permission of the publisher. The use of short quotations or occasional page copying for not-for-profit activities such as personal or group study is permitted and encouraged provided proper credit is included by providing publication title and author name with each use.

ISBN 978-0-9896997-0-9

LCCN 2013946075

Published by ToDoBlue Press

206-763-6800

Editing and layout by Allie Gillebo
Cover design by Dave Hewer
Author photos by Ethan Breitling, Jeremy Echols & Justin Gillebo

Printed in the United States of America
For Worldwide Distribution

CONTENTS

Foreword

Jerrod Sessler has been a fellow promoter of healthy eating, juicing and living well for over a decade now. Our friendship began when my movie, *Fat, Sick & Nearly Dead*, was released in the US in 2010. Jerrod felt strongly about my cause and was a huge supporter of the film. Since then, we've shared stories and encouraged others to make the changes to pursue the lifestyle they deserve.

Jerrod's journey is one filled with gritty determination. In 1999, Jerrod was diagnosed with a life threatening form of cancer: a stage IV metastasized melanoma. Jerrod was told it was unlikely he would live much longer, and had just a five percent chance of survival. Rather than shattering his dreams, Jerrod took this as an opportunity to make them come true. One of those dreams was to start a family with his best friend and wife, Nikki. Some years later, I can tell you first hand that they not only have a beautiful family, but also are a model of good health. These guys are a perfect example of the benefits of a healthy lifestyle and provide inspiration for those on their own journey to improved wellbeing. Jerrod's second love is racing, and he's spent plenty of time on the NASCAR circuit – and is teaching this art to his kids, who will never be late for school again.

The healthy choices Jerrod makes every day have not only given the Sessler family a fantastic healthy foundation on which to build a happy life, but have inspired other families to follow in their path. We are talking about simple, everyday changes that anybody can achieve – as basic as eating the right foods, juicing, and exercising regularly.

Food Chains is all about living the good life. I don't mean the Hollywood "good life", or the something for nothing "good life", but the real life good life--where you get back what you put in. Jerrod's personal experience of celebrating fantastic victories and surviving the toughest of challenges, only to come out the other side juicing and smiling, makes him an inspiring advocate. *Food Chains* is not only packed with practical, useful information to help you to achieve your own goals; it also provides a deeper insight into the experiences of someone who has walked the walk. I hope you draw inspiration from Jerrod's story, and use this book as a companion on your own journey to wellbeing and personal health. Jerrod has motivated me and I know he can do the same for you.

— Joe Cross, founder of Reboot with Joe and creator of *Fat, Sick & Nearly Dead.*

Introduction

I'm excited to be able to share my story with you, but even more excited to know that it will encourage you to look more closely at your own winning story!

The purpose of this book is to illuminate the real bondage (chains) that we live with due to the challenges associated with modern-day food masquerading as nutritious.

This is also a celebration, for me, of living through a diagnosis that could have been a death sentence and to share the things I've learned. If you are searching for answers, you will find the contents of this book encouraging and enlightening.

I realize that book introductions are something often skimmed or skipped, so let me simply say that the book is organized first with an overview of my story so you can gain familiarity with how I achieved health; then I discuss the dilemma with our food and how we choose to shackle ourselves with food chains; and finally, I lay out a specific plan for change and health for you to readily implement.

Now, let's start breaking some chains!

CHAPTER ONE

My Chains That Led To Cancer

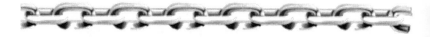

My story is miraculous. Doctors gave me a slim chance, a sliver really, of being alive to write this book. Thankfully, miracles do happen and your story can have a happy ending too!

I am deeply passionate about a few things in life. Thinking on a grand scale and expecting big things to happen, I rarely live in "the now" because I am planning for the future. I choose to be present with my family, but I admit to being easily disappointed if I don't anticipate the circumstances I face. This may help shed some light on what a terminal diagnosis at the age of twenty-nine was like for me. I had already planned out the next couple of decades and I certainly didn't want to miss out on them. Little did I know I would indeed get to live long into the future, but my path didn't align at all with what I planned prior to the diagnosis.

If we ever have the opportunity to meet, don't spend nearly as much time with me as you do with my wife, Nikki. She is one of the wonders of the world. Nikki is simply a wonderful, incredible, beautiful, talented and loving person. Together, we have three great kids that I will talk a bit more about later. My family is truly one of my greatest treasures. You may be surprised, however, to learn of the challenges we faced together in our relationship with food.

There is a tendency in all of us in the western culture to live to eat. Think about it. When was the last time you attended a social event that didn't involve food—most likely unhealthy food? Our gatherings seem to be an excuse to outdo each other, and most people scoff at the thought of healthiness in our choices. Food manufacturers and establishments have the upper hand by twisting our taste buds with flavor additives that are addictive and harmful. Everyone keeps raising the bar in terms of flavor excitement so we have in essence, as a culture, driven these companies to use more and more of these deadly, disease-creating additives. One of my great concerns for the long-term health of our nation is the dangerous food additives in processed foods. The use of them is rampant and the results are devastating.

While living in Seattle, Washington in 1998, Nikki and I began a journey that was founded in our mutual faith and desire for adventure in our lives. We both quit our corporate jobs and started Hope4Youth, a non-profit organization dedicated to encouraging young people. We also started a little construction company. At that time I was actively enjoying the experience of my racing dreams by participating in a regional NASCAR series.

My preferred sport is auto racing and I have been in pursuit of my racing dreams since I was a toddler. When I was only four, I told my mom that I wanted to drive racecars. I have always been competitive and loved speed. As a kid, I enjoyed bicycles, go-carts, motorcycles, and as I got older, full-sized NASCAR racecars.

Along with racing, another pursuit of mine is the illumination of truth and the never-ending chase to fully understand it. Truth is the foundation for all ethics, beliefs, motives, and wisdom. It is never moving and stays constant forever. It's the basis for my understanding of life and the world that we live in. I will never know everything there is to know, but education helps me continue to grow and understand the framework in which we live.

It is a great honor to provide a place for truth to reside and to impact the world around me. It is an additional honor to be alive and able to share with you the things that I have learned.

It is often hard to really believe that a few years ago I was facing a very serious cancer diagnosis. Nikki and I were enjoying life. We were growing in our marriage, our business was flourishing, and we felt like our lives were positively impacting our community. Sometime during 1997, however, I noticed a mole on my back; it was itchy at times, discolored and irregularly shaped. I visited the doctor for a racing physical and he said not to worry about it, because it didn't seem like anything to cause concern.

In late 1999, my mom, who was a nurse, grew tired of watching me back up against wall corners to scratch the mole. She scheduled an appointment with a dermatologist. One look and the mole was removed. Tissue samples that were sent for analysis revealed malignant melanoma cancer, and I quickly found myself at a specialized cancer care clinic with very little understanding of my options for healing.

At the clinic, they did a sentinel node biopsy—a test to determine where the cancer was exactly. They needed to know if it had metastasized, or spread throughout my body. At age twenty-nine, sitting in the doctor's office with a lead ball in my stomach, I listened as I was diagnosed with advanced metastasized melanoma, a serious skin cancer that had already spread throughout my body by the lymphatic system. The doctors gave me a five percent chance of living past my thirties with no treatment, and up to a twenty percent chance of doing so with medical treatment. Neither of these options held a lot of promise.

A quick search on metastasized melanoma will reveal that it is a very serious form of cancer, contributing to around two percent of all cancer deaths annually. Metastatic melanoma in particular means that the cancer has spread, commonly via the lymphatic system, from the original location. To date, there is no known tracking mechanism other than inflamed (enlarged) lymph nodes or a tumor that is at least the size of a dime. Therefore, it is difficult for a patient to know if the cancer is gone or simply growing in the background until it reveals itself again. Melanoma tends to wreak even more havoc during a subsequent bout because it has had time to spread into multiple locations; it grows generally unnoticed until it is of significant size.

My discussions with oncologists centered on treatment options, including taking the drug Interferon, well known for its toxic side effects. I must mention here that one of the toxic side effects of Interferon is that about five percent of the people who take it actually die from the drug itself. Other slightly more palatable options included participating in a double blind, two-year cancer study, not knowing if I was receiving a sugar pill or the new experimental medication. Another option was chemotherapy, to achieve what one doctor called a "clean sweep of your system." The whole "clean sweep" terminology really tipped me over. It doesn't sound so odd now, and I guess it got their point across, but it certainly didn't help me to agree to the treatment or feel any more comfortable about their true understanding of what we were fighting. The doctors were quite abrupt when mentioning that Nikki and I would probably never have children, and that I was done racing.

To understand how devastating this news was, you first must know a little bit more about Nikki and me. When Nikki was a little girl, she had dolls and dreamed of one day being the mother of her own wonderful little babies. She dressed them, cared for them and loved on them as she does with our beautiful children now. I don't think I need to dig any deeper into my dream box to demonstrate what "not ever racing again" meant to me. This was an earth-shattering and unacceptable life theme for us. The idea of taking these two passions from us was simply not an option for our futures, based on everything we had ever dreamed about.

Nikki and I had spent a day with my uncle and aunt in Chicago two years before, during the summer of 1997. The company and relationships were wonderful, but mostly we were perplexed about their eating habits and lifestyle. They were really dogmatic about what they ate and very inflexible. They stuck with raw produce, salads, juices, etc. They could not eat anything (so it seemed) and of course, at that time, we would eat just about anything. As we have grown, we have come to realize the gap was a combination of culture, age, wisdom and maturity.

As for their eating habits, my aunt had suffered from multiple sclerosis many years earlier but lived a healthy life while eating their unconventional diet. This day turned out to be providential for us because it was the experience we recalled when I was diagnosed. We got a copy of the video titled How to Eliminate Sickness, (now called God's Ultimate Way to Health), by Rev. George Malkmus, Lit.D.. Our entire family and a small contingent of friends gathered around the television at my sister's home on Christmas Day in 1999 to watch this video, and the results deeply changed the course of our lives. In my case, it was like I had gone from sleeping very deeply under a tombstone to living an exciting, vibrant, world-changing life. We believe the message we heard resonated as truth and that we were blessed by the knowledge. We set out to learn what we could and change what we had to. And change we did.

Some of the doctors were willing to work with us on a monitored program that would identify if the cancer spread, returned, or grew in other regions. I visited a dermatologist, a surgeon, and received a CAT scan at regular intervals for two years.

The oncologist made it clear, with an affronted tirade, that he wanted nothing to do with us. I feel bad that so many doctors do not actually understand how very simple the path to health and healing can be. I feel even worse that our culture trains us to hold these fallible doctors up on a pedestal that requires them to achieve results above the capabilities they in fact can actually achieve.

I enjoy taking calls from doctors inquiring about the results of my self-treatment. If their sole purpose is assisting people to achieve health and healing, then their course will differ from conventional modalities. Doctors need to build relationships with their patients, understand them, and track with them as coaches as they traverse various ailments.

Within months of implementing the diet changes I will discuss later in the book, the doctors were amazed that things looked so great and asked us what we were doing. After two years, I decided to discontinue the CAT scans due to their absolute toxic side effects. Every time I went in there, I had to drink the nasty shake needed for the machine to see my insides as I passed through the scanner. I couldn't take just a little sip of it either. They had this super-sized cup that they kept topping off. I drank until I must have consumed a half-gallon. I began to think about how closely we had learned to watch what we were putting into our bodies and how interesting it was that the doctors were not required to show me the ingredient list on this "shake."

So, I made a little mini-mission out of discovering what actually was in the mystery shake. Imagine my surprise when even the doctors had no clue what the shake contained but still insisted it was safe to drink. After all, it was a medical thing! It had to be safe, right? After obtaining the ingredient list directly from the manufacturer, I found out it was full of excitotoxins. This shows what a little bit of education can mean for you in every day life. Learning is the key to taking control of your health.

In addition to drinking that horrible shake each time I went into the machine, they also injected a horrible clear substance into my blood. I found something quite interesting but not at all enjoyable as part of this injection. Within milliseconds after they started the injection, my rectum would literally feel like it was on fire. How on earth did that junk travel through my arm, into my heart and get pumped all the way down to my behind in milliseconds? Even more importantly, why did it feel like that? After a few of those, I just felt like whatever was going into me was worse than just keeping track of my own health by the way I felt and the signals from my body.

As I transitioned my diet and lifestyle, I began to really get more in touch with what my body liked and what it didn't like, and this knowledge really became helpful to me as I defined what I would and would not ingest. To this day, I use this same approach, which over time, becomes even more valuable. I could do a lot more damage more quickly to myself by eating unhealthy foods now than when my intestines were coated with a layer of fat, mucus, and bile. This layer somewhat shielded my organs from many of the toxins I used to eat but the overall lifestyle caused myriad other problems.

From the time we started, it took us about three months to clear out the food we had, and we struggled with what to do with many of the items. We gave some to the needy, threw a lot away, and ate the rest ourselves. I started drinking thirty-two ounces of carrot juice each day, and taking three tablespoons of a dehydrated green powder from barley. We immediately stopped eating all dairy and meat products and ate a lot of salads. In the first three months I lost forty pounds, and by the sixth year I was sitting at about sixty pounds under my previous weight. I was close to what Dr. Fuhrman (author of Eat To Live) suggests is a healthy weight for a man my size. I feel better than I've ever felt in my life.

Like you, I really do enjoy food. I don't feel deprived EVER! Seriously, I really enjoy what I am eating and know that what I am eating is more satisfying and more fulfilling, not to mention healthier, than what anyone is eating on the standard western diet. If you are interested in what I am eating today then ask me. Connect with me and ask me any day. I will share what I am eating today!

The blessings of living a healthy lifestyle continue to this day. We now have three incredible kids—Gabe (2001), Farrell (2003) and Jake (2005). They all love fresh veggies and fruit, and want nothing to do with candy or other junk most kids their age crave. Each of them started getting the dehydrated green powder on their pacifier as young as three months. Each morning, for years, we made a mix of this with water. I prefer mine in water as a little juice starter for the day but all of the kids get a bit of each on a spoon and they love it. More recently, we have transitioned more to juicing greens and making green smoothies regularly. We feel the freshness and taste of this to be superior to the rehydrated solutions. We do however still use the powder as a backup resource.

In general, none of the children have ever been sick or required drugs. The boys have had some occasions when they have over-eaten. Those proved to be our first and only "up at night" experience for our family. It is simply their body refusing the junk they put in it or even just too much of a good thing. Sure, they have fallen out of bed or wet the bed here and there, but for the most part, they have slept through the night from a couple months of age. I mention this because I think our diet and their "levelness" plays a huge role in the overall success and stability of our family. I can't imagine the stress and strain of sickness in children and all the implications of that including, but not limited to, being up at night, fatigue (for Nikki and/or I as well as the kids), bad attitudes, and unclear thinking.

Nikki and I traveled to a health-training seminar in Sacramento, California, during the summer of 2002. The training was focused on educating people like us who desire to learn more about living a healthy diet and lifestyle and to help others do the same. We have taught hundreds of classes through the years on lifestyle basics and food preparation. I love to share my passion and, unlike my wife, I also enjoy public speaking on topics for which I have great passion. Nikki is really interesting to listen to, however, and if someone really wants to hear her she will speak as well. Because of this I began to take on speaking engagements on the subjects of health and business ethics and, of course, some racing stories get sprinkled into the mix. We launched the Hope4Health Foundation to support our training efforts.

One of the tools we developed in conjunction with the help of a Naturopath and Wellness Research Scientist is available on our web site at www.hope4health.org. This tool allows you to measure your health potential by answering a few simple questions. To do so, click on "Take the PerforMax Challenge." We launched an organic produce delivery service called Freggies (www.freggies.com) in 2006. The purpose of Freggies is chiefly to get fresh, organic produce into the hands of as many people as possible at a good price, and secondly, to enable others who desire to follow in our path in teaching and leading to build relationships with people locally. I have a long-term vision for planting "health cafés" through ventures like HACO TACO (www.hacotaco.com) and Good2Go Café (www.good2gocafe.com) as well. These are intended to be a part of the solution to the overwhelming health care issues that our culture is facing.

As the years passed by, we continued to look at every aspect of our lives for areas where we could make some gains health-wise. I began to look at our lives as if they were on a scale—one side was toxic intake and the other was nutritional intake. For example, if we drink tap water we are adding to both sides of the scale because there are toxins in the water, but of course, some benefit as well. So, it made sense to start drinking distilled water with liquid minerals added back to it. Another example is the soaps we use in our home. Everything from body soap to laundry soap and every kind of cleaner in between was reviewed. We set up an account with Melaleuca and have really enjoyed their products as well as many others offered through Hallelujah Acres. We also purchased a very good quality air cleaner. I am still in awe at how clear the air is on a sunny day with the sun shining through a window or skylight. No more air floaties!

There are other things to think about, such as building products. Kids' play centers, fences, and outdoor furniture are often built with highly chemically-saturated building products that protect the wood and make it last longer but the chemicals are very toxic to the body. If you like the fancy foam mattresses and pillows that have become mainstream the last few years, be careful. We open ours and let it sit in the garage for at least a few weeks (preferably a few months) before we put it on our bed. That gives them a chance to air out some of the toxins left over from the manufacturing process.

One of the best things I have noticed about living this lifestyle is how much clearer I think. I just have significantly more mental clarity. All of my relationships are better. Communication is better. I make better decisions, which impacts everything I do. I have been blessed to be able to use my position as a cancer survivor, leader, NASCAR driver, businessman, husband, and father as a platform to help spread the good news in many ways.

One of the people I met after I began this journey was Bill. Bill was in his late fifties and had contracted hepatitis C about twenty-five years prior. He had struggled with poor results from the various approaches and modalities of the medical community for many years. Finally one day, he heard that changing his lifestyle could have an effect on the hepatitis C symptoms. The lifestyle changes he learned were similar in nature to what we have done. After just a few weeks, he experienced amazing results--so much so that he found himself riddled with fear. To Bill, it was just too much of a good thing. This may seem like an odd reaction, but it was quite true and real for him. He had achieved a level of mental clarity that he had never felt before and the experience was possibly like some sort of mental high.

He found that he could increase this feeling by the way he ate and by how much fresh juice he drank, along with other diet changes. He found that the full level of clarity was too much for him to be comfortable with, so he backed it down with cooked foods or pasteurized juices rather than raw or fresh juice. I would agree that there is a mental fog that seems to lift when I eat healthfully, but I never experienced a fear from the clarity like Bill did. I believe my personality thrives on such clarity while others may be overwhelmed or even desire a bit of ambiguity. I further wonder how much our spiritual lives play into this. Maybe Bill was seeing things that he had just not ever been taught to understand.

I am grateful for the growing relationship I have with many people in the real health community, which includes the extended family of people that we have met, helped, been helped by, and just generally been overjoyed to be associated with. Many of these people will do whatever it takes to help people understand how to become healthy and how to stay that way.

All of us have an uphill battle to overcome the passivity and apathy towards on-going education. For some reason in our culture, interest in education is just not common. Our culture is filled with people who want to consume the moment without a care for the future. Most of us are more concerned about our status in society than the number of days we will actually get to enjoy that status. Unhealthy meals entertain us for the moment, but cumulatively cost us up to fifty percent of our life. Knowing this, then do they really taste that good? Life generally begins to shut down, or at least show significant downward trends, at the age of fifty. Sure, many people exist beyond that age but are they really living? They are limited in their activities due to their physical ailments or due to their prescribed drug regime. More on this later, but for now let me just make one more point: Have you ever considered how you learn? I know that I enjoy learning by doing. As I have gotten older, I find that I also enjoy reading books and filling my days with meaningful thought and consideration of concepts that I don't fully understand. How do you learn? It is disappointing to me that we don't appoint more time to education. We see K-12 as the requirement, rather than the prerequisite, to a life of learning. I believe our elementary years are simply a time for us to learn the basics and to understand how we learn individually. It is likely that those of you who are reading this book think in similar terms because you have taken the time to open this book, so maybe you agree that education should be honored.

I believe in you. I know you can do anything with your life that you set out to do. If you are faced with a situation like I was or you have other issues going on, consider what you learn here, and what preconceived ideas you may have due to misinformation you have adopted as you work through the balance of this book.

CHAPTER TWO

Who Are You?

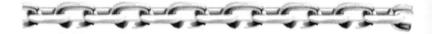

I am personally persuaded to believe that there is a great and mighty God and that this God did actually create us. Because of that, I also have certain core questions that can only be answered by analyzing with a clear perspective of what God's intention was with creation and for the nourishment of creation.

If you disagree or find yourself offended that I would suggest there is a connection between our health and a creator then please take my request to read this chapter with an open heart and mind in search of truth. I feel it is important to have a framework for the original intent if we want to successfully land on a complete solution to the problems keeping us in chains.

Food is a wonderful gift and a well-conceived plan for the nourishment of our bodies. It is a life-sustaining tool. We are in error when we esteem food beyond what it is designed to be as nourishment. The result of this is a false elevation of a material thing to a roll where it begins to take control over us. We put ourselves in chains by viewing our food as something more than the tool that it is.

We tend to fall in love with our food. We allow it to control our circumstances, our moods, and us. We give it control over our minds in subtle ways. We do this regularly and it is called gluttony.

Gluttony is the act of giving yourself over to your food. We literally put our food in control to a certain extent. Depending upon the culture gluttony is seen as either a vice or a status symbol. The relative affluence of the culture affects this view in both ways. The wealthy may take pride in the security of having plenty, and may be prone to show it off, but may be faced with the results of social backlash when confronted with the less fortunate.

Gluttony according to Wikipedia:

"Gluttony, derived from the Latin *gluttire*, meaning 'to gulp down or swallow,' means over-indulgence and over-consumption of food, drink, or intoxicants to the point of waste. In some Christian denominations, it is considered one of the seven deadly sins—a misplaced desire of food or its withholding from the needy."

So when do we reach the line of acceptable indulgence? After all, we want to know when we have crossed over it, right? Furthermore, it perplexes me to think we can't go out and have a nice meal with family and enjoy eating whatever we want as much as we want. My advice is that we should attempt to live according to our needs and occasionally indulge, provided it does not harm others or ourselves. So what does that look like practically in my life? I don't live for food. Food is a tool; but, there are some that are simply too wonderful, divine, and nearly indescribable to not indulge. I believe we should enjoy these times and remain very reasonable about our consumption on a day-to-day basis.

I want to begin by simply laying a foundation that food is not the problem, but the love of food (gluttony) is a problem.

Gluttony is universal and pervasive. It would be difficult to find even one among us who has not succumbed to the taunts of gluttony. Gluttony can even manifest in many forms outside of the context of food. Here are some examples of how it threatens our peace and joy:

Impatience. Eating before it is time and never letting yourself feel a bit of hunger. This is solely out of habit, due to the pleasing of the palate or physical self, and is contrary to what we know and believe about where our full satisfaction should come from. I feel best on an empty stomach or with a slight ache for some nourishment. As a culture we fear this place and so we stay far from it.

I Deserve The Best. We seek delicacies and enormous flavors. The birth of excitotoxins is the solution for our endless yearning for more flavors. We see shows of people who travel the world looking for, tasting, and taking pleasure from the very best of foods. It is not that we should deprive ourselves of these wonderful, nourishing foods; but the never-satisfied palate is dangerous.

Additions or Stimulants. Similar to any addictive substance, food is one that brings pleasures mentally and physically. There are literally hundreds of unnatural flavorings that are used in food or sold as a seasoning in an attempt to fulfill this desire. Dr. Russell Blaylock explains excitotoxins, the role they play in food, and the diseases they are contributing towards in his book entitled, *Excitotoxins*.

Seconds Please. We have a restaurant near that serves good quality food, but their claim to fame is the size of their plates. Our family could easily feed from a single plate, yet it is common to see each person order their own and do a decent job of clearing it. We find comfort in a full table, belly, and bank account. Quantity is one of the easiest forms of gluttony to grasp. We all have a voracious appetite for more.

Live To Eat. We tend to approach food with an excessive desire. We get very excited about eating and the prospect of food. We rarely meet for the sake of meeting, but more commonly for the excuse of eating. We are simply too eager for our next meal. I have a friend who told a story of how his father always talked about the contents of the next meal while at the table eating.

Food is fun and should be enjoyed, but it is clear from these items that we take it where it is not intended to go. Why is the gluttony of food so pervasive?

A friend recently helped me to understand this more clearly. He is a self-diagnosed "gluttoner", overweight and burdened with the results physically, mentally, and spiritually of his choices on a daily basis. While we were catching up recently, he asked if I knew why gluttony was so difficult to overcome. Of course I was glad to listen. What he described made sense and came from a perspective I had not ever realized prior to that conversation.

It is expected that in close-knit relationships we will talk about the struggles we face in our lives. Often inappropriate sexual desires or habits bubble to the top. It isn't as common that we address or face the socially acceptable habits openly with our friends. For example, the way we use our time, money, or food. Talking about the more pervasive or embarrassing habits doesn't happen as easily or as often.

My friend pointed out that we could easily coach someone close to us on the negative effects of pornography, gambling, adultery, smoking, or cutting. Food, on the other hand, is a different challenge because we can't just avoid food altogether. In fact, it may be the only common tool we cannot avoid all together that leads the majority of us, if not all of us, into obsession.

If all of this talk of gluttony just seems over the top then set aside your food for a few days and limit yourself to just fresh raw vegetables and fruit or juice from either or both. If you can do that for a few days and not have any negative effects then maybe you are one of the few people on the planet who do not have a problem with gluttony.

The warning here is similar to many examples we see and read about. Continuing to indulge in a harmful behavior over a lifetime simply indicates the severity of struggle we are caught up in as we seek food, comfort, wealth, and control over anything else.

Similar to my previous comments about elevating or too highly esteeming our food giving it control over us, we can also do the same with our obedience to the so called *right* food. What I mean is that we can become prideful about our success with or over food. This too can be an unhealthy trap and one that I have certainly dipped into a time or two myself.

We tend to worship created things instead of the Creator God. Food is a tool provided by the Creator. Food is part of this creation. It is not the Creator and should not be worshiped in any form or manner. We will achieve success in overcoming our food idolizing by first actively seeing what we are doing and then taking steps to correct it. One helpful step is to write down your priorities. What is more important than food? Of course, it gets confusing because we need food to live, but the act of actively questioning it causes us to see our food as the fuel tool that it really is. It may be momentary and may seem like a never-ending challenge, but it is most certainly possible.

The most important thing I have found in being able to successfully avoid the horrible food habits that plague our culture is not a stoic focus on that habit as you might assume. There is a much simpler path but it is not readily apparent. What is most important to me is to understand who I am, what I am, who created me, why I am here, and what my greatest mission is in life.

When I think like this then I am able to respond properly to many things in life instead of the obvious approach, which may look a lot like box checking or self-discipline. I am an engineer, so I tend to have fairly square corners. I like accuracy and strive for perfection—even though I am learning perfection is a myth. Therefore, I wrongly tend to lean towards the attempt at self-discipline instead of simply recognizing who I am.

So, who are you? What are you here for? Whose are you? Have you ever thought through these sort of questions? I would encourage you to do so. Knowing the answers to these vital questions helps us understand and transform us on a moment-by-moment basis through our days?.

How can we capture success in our diet by understanding who we are? At the core, knowing who we are and why we exist means that everything is about who we are rather than what we do. Clearly, this understanding enables complete freedom from shame, fear and worry. We recognize our position in life and we begin to focus on what we can and should do rather than how we can fall in love with a material item like food.

To better understand what I am talking about, think about the traditional five senses: sight, hearing, touch, smell, and taste. What would you eat if you could not taste anything? Seriously, what would you eat? I think I would choose something that felt good in my mouth, or maybe something that smelled good as I was eating it. Maybe I'd choose something that simply looked divine. Well, what if we took away taste and smell? Now all you could do is look at the food, feel it going down, and I guess, listen to whatever it sounds like to eat it or prepare it.

If we allow enough time to pass, and we follow this line of thinking far enough, we will find that we would be eating the things that cost the least. We have food manufacturers filled with talented people today that are forced to work within the bounds of our senses as they attempt to create irresistible products. Their jobs would be so much easier if all they had to do was create a thing that looked wonderful, didn't kill us instantly, and was super cheap!

I believe we are made to enjoy our food but not to fall in love with it. If we do then we will not eat junk that is not nourishing and we would enjoy the satisfaction of feeling great all the time. So go bite into and enjoy a super juicy, sweet, organic red pepper!

Don't Mess With My Food

Is it now a bit clearer why we avoid the discussion of the gluttony of food? It is common to hear a teacher mention food in a list of bad habits that we adopt, but rarely will they dig any deeper. The truth is that they simply don't know very much about gluttony in food, and they are most likely just as deep into it as those they are charged to lead. Furthermore, this isn't really the proper role for a most teachers, and those who do teach it realize how socially unacceptable it would be to discuss.

Like many other quality teachings, some focus should be invested and promoted in the area of gluttony of food. It is clearly a piece of the message for us to learn. Unfortunately, there are an enormous number of people who are stricken with the results of limited understanding. The struggles and challenges we see daily shared throughout social media demonstrates the magnitude of our ignorance in the area of gluttony.

Occasionally I get negative emails, phone calls, voice mails, and letters. People will criticize my perspective in their blogs, on the news, and in print. One of the most recent threats I got via voice mail indicated, using the choicest words, that my position on health care (which, by the way, should be called "disease care") was wrong. I wonder if this person has spent a quarter of their life learning, studying, and putting into practice the truths about diet and lifestyle and see the impact on our health? As I listened to the voice mail, two things came to mind that I believe, in hearing, would have changed his mind. First, forcing companies to pay for disease care will drive salaries down in an equal proportion; and second, telling entrepreneurs how to spend their profits will kill the entire free market system that our country thrives upon. I am always interested in debating these maters with anyone who is open to discussion.

Another time, an employee literally got in my face, and was yelling at me and accusing me of heresy because of my teaching in the area of nutrition. I got the smattering of saliva with the finger in my chest from this distraught individual. I feel bad for this person to this day. I hurt for him because he is so ignorant of the bigger truth that is so much greater and deeper than anything to do with food.

I love food. I enjoy food. I take great pleasure in playing in the kitchen, but I ultimately see food as a tool. It is a necessary tool for me to continue to live!

Ultimately, food is not the problem, but what we do with our food, and our desire and love of food is the problem.

Original Intent

What is our food? Seriously, what is food? What is ideal and why? Is there an ideal for all of us or just for some?

As I get older, I have increasing respect for those current and past who contemplated deep questions. It seems many of us choose to consume life without questions, rather than living life by questioning. To be clear, I have never considered myself to be much of a thinker (i.e. smart), but I do like to question things and then dig for answers. I have added a lot of color to my life using this approach, and I know I am much closer to knowing truth in various areas because I question, question, question until I feel that I understand the real answers. I suppose I am a bit like Josh, played by Tom Hanks and David Moscow, in the movie Big (1988) a comedy about a young boy trapped in a man's body. While in conference with colleagues of the toy company where he worked he was confronted about his inability to understand. He simply says, "I don't get it" as they bantered a marketing scheme for a toy that he didn't think would be the least bit interesting to kids. The key is that he stood up and said he didn't understand something.

Here's where I want to challenge you. What is the meaning of life? Don't stop reading, I will make this quick. You will be better off for it and, like a good trial lawyer, I will tie this all back together soon.

What is the meaning of life? Have you ever thought about it? I mean for more than seven seconds until something less taxing hits your brain. Get a yellow note pad out and write down a question, then just begin making notes about what comes to mind. Or, if you want a quick answer based on someone else's yellow note pad time, just peruse the answers on the Internet.

Here is why I think I am here: *To submit to God and to enjoy life.*

There is a lot more to this, of course, but the main points are as follows. I believe God created us, which is important to recognize that in the context of attempting to get free of the voluntary (and unnecessary) chains we put on ourselves in this life. I also believe that God intends us to be filled with joy even though it is often hard to see in our circumstances.

Now let's tie the basic framework of the meaning of life to what we eat.

If I am to submit to God and to live a joyful existence then can I best do that through proper or improper treatment of my physical body?

I think the answer is obvious, so lets dig into why it seems so difficult to execute.

Each day, we toss multiple questions over to our subconscious where a decision is made, which affects our choices, attitude, and outcome of our lives. All of this happens without us even consciously realizing it. So, what we truly believe about life really does have a lot of control over the outcome of our lives. I would describe this as our worldview. What we believe—not what we say we believe, but what we truly believe—has an impact on every one of our actions and decisions. Therefore, it is of first importance to know what you believe. Again, not what you say you believe, but what you truly believe. If you don't know then just look back at your choices, which will indicate what you believe in your heart. If you do look, and you don't like what you see, then you are on a wonderful new path of determining how you change what you truly believe into what you really want to believe. That is one of life's biggest challenges, and sadly only very few stand on the question long enough to figure it out. I hope you enjoy this adventure. Big questions like this will help you to shift and mold your future into a more joyful experience.

I am not fun to be around when I am not feeling well. It has been years since anyone has had to deal with this, but I remember days long ago when I could be demanding and just plain difficult if I didn't feel well. Eating right, getting good sleep, exercising regularly, mitigating stress, and managing my priorities all contribute to me truly living what I believe to be truth. The times when I don't make the right choice in these areas, I realize I am taking something away from myself and my family and friends.

Living as healthy of a lifestyle as possible enables me to focus on the bigger picture and not myself. That is not to say living and eating healthy is a magic pill for a better life. I do believe I notice an additional clarity of mind and seemingly clearer thought processes, but that should not be a surprise. If my body is in shape and not feeling ill, then I am less likely to actually be thinking about it. If I am not thinking about my body, then I am less likely to be focused on it.

"UNCLE"

After reading this far (and especially if this is your first introduction to this information) you may be about to cry out "uncle," as if to say you give up and you want it to stop. Some who read this may feel this way while others enjoy it as a breath of fresh air. Each of us will wonder, at some point, why we face the things we do physically or otherwise. This question comes directly from our own personal perspective on who we are and why we exist. My encouragement is to ponder—but never doubt—that there is an epic story in which each of us is just a small part.

CHAPTER THREE

Shackles

Have you ever wondered why we need to eat?

I am an engineer at heart and by training, so questions like this lead me to a barrage of additional questions, such as:

- If we are *supposed* to eat something then what is that something?

- More importantly, is that something already here or is it still being crafted in the food factories and warehouses of the world?

- If it is not yet here then who is going to create the perfect food that fully satisfies, in every way possible , (such as smell, texture, taste, versatility, convenience, and of course, health benefits)?

- If it is already here, can we improve it? Or, should we be messing with it at all?

- If it is already here then what motivates people and companies to assemble teams to work tirelessly to create and package a mixture of the available resources and to sell this substance as food?

- If that is happening then who is behind the closed door of the labs verifying that what is actually put into these concoctions is in fact a food substance?

- And even deeper into the rabbit hole, who sets the standard or draws the line on what is acceptable in terms of ingredients to use when crafting and assembling these laboratory creations?

This line of thinking could be debated and discussed for months – even years. My point with taking you on this journey is the fact that your presupposition to these very questions establishes your framework for what size, color, and type of food chains you daily shackle yourself as you view your food. These are your food chains. In this book, I want to help you get free!

Wouldn't it be helpful if you could see how your personal food chains are defining your expectations? This is an incredible, frightening thing to consider. What I am asking is, how do the lies that you believe limit the life that you live? And the life that you *will* live. How do you get yourself to a place where you are even willing to have an argument with yourself in an effort to discover what you believe that is actually false?

For obvious reasons I am going to limit this just to the relationship between our food and our potential. The larger consideration is certainly for our entire lives, however; our falsities are actually grossly limiting our experience and our expression of this wonderful and amazing thing called life!

The problem is not in finding answers. Everyone has a sea of information in front of himself or herself – especially today. Sure, one could argue that there is too much information and it is all so confusing. I would agree to an extent, but a fairly small amount of effort to ferret out the truth is relatively quick and painless in most situations. The point is that the answers are out there and they are readily available. The problem is the act of implementation of those truths once they are unearthed. Why is it so difficult to see the answers *and* the path to implementation?

Philosophically, one could argue that the question does not matter. If a person is happy where they are at and they do not have a greater vision then an education for them would actually ruin their current blissful sense of completeness. This is in fact true, but it also must be understood that a person living like this is also going to only experience a small portion of the joy that is ultimately possible in their lives. Sure, they are joyful for a while; but eventually it becomes mundane and even a burden to keep up with the daily requirements of their station. If only they had a great vision that allowed them to expand their thinking.

Back to reality. Most of us know we are not hitting the ball out of the park in regards to our diet and lifestyle. We know we are believing lies and we swallow them hook, line, and sinker because they taste good and we believe they won't actually have an adverse effect on our health over the long term.

Thankfully you are reading this book, which is a great sign that you are willing to ask yourself some hard questions. When you reach for 'x', what causes you to do that? Why do you believe that is good for you? Why do you feel you can't live without it, even though you know it isn't good for you? At what point will you be ready to walk away forever and not feel like you are depriving yourself?

I will spend the rest of this book, and my life, attempting to answer the big implementation question for myself with my food chains and with other shackles I choose to put on myself. Through my experiences, I will share with you and others what I have learned, what has worked, and what has not. Much of that is included in this book and, although I feel like I have traveled most of this path already, I may likely have entire new corridors opened for me in the future that I need to traverse. It is encouraging for me to know that I will be doing it with you too as I face these questions and challenges.

CHAPTER FOUR

Why Do I Do That?

On the way to our favorite Mexican restaurant I began to daydream about the meal ahead. *I really enjoy the veggie fajitas but hope they don't come out overcooked or greasy. What will the kids and Nikki order? Will we get corn or flour tortillas? I wish they had some really great romaine or butter leaf lettuce that we could use as wraps instead. How can I control myself with the free chips they offer as an appetizer?* I agree to just not have any chips. I know I can't control the volume, so why have any at all? They are not good for me and they fill my stomach with empty calories.

When we arrive, I catch a smell of the food, the chips, and quickly toss my best intentions out the window. It is *just* a meal. It is *just* this time. It is *just* a few chips. What is the big deal? Eat on!

I am going to stop and get a donut. They offer a free one to every visitor so I will just be in-and-out. I can taste it already. I don't even like donuts but something about these is appealing so much so that I am willing to risk the results with a quick stop to get just one. I am also willing to sacrifice whatever the result will be on and in my body, which can't be that good, right? After all, it is *just* one donut.

I arrive and quickly realize, I am on my way to the office and it is early in the week so all of the staff and some guests will be there so I should just grab a dozen to share with them. And, of course I get the free one too to justify the cost of the dozen more because I get a baker's dozen for the same price!

Within a few minutes down the highway, half the box is in my stomach and I am trying to decide if I should take half the box in and admit I could not stop at just one or should I just eat the other half as well? I already feel terrible so how much worse can I feel if I just eat the rest?

I got a pint of my favorite flavor of ice cream. It is Almond Joy, which I call A-Joy for short. Justin, the owner of Full Tilt ice cream shop, texts me occasionally when he knows it is in production so I know to stop by in the next few days. This week I stopped and bought three pints of various flavors. They are all vegan so I feel good about being able to enjoy a cultural staple treat with the kids without the implications and horrible physical effects of the dairy and chemicals. But, I need to consume it within reason because it is still loaded with sweeteners that won't do any good for me – especially if I consume them in excess.

I get home and get the ice cream pints into the freezer, but we pull them out later that evening during a break in the movie we are watching. I scoop some for the family based on their choosing and decide I will just have a bite or two out of the pint while we resume the movie. Even though my mouth is frozen and I essentially stop sensing the real flavors after the first few bites, I continue and consume the entire pint.

It is super hot today. I need to get some cold water. Wait—there is a drive thru right up here a couple of minutes. Boy, an ice-cold soda sure *sounds like a quencher right now. I could down two of them! I should not stop however as I do have a problem with it and I have been trying to stop drinking sugary drinks for quite a while. I have cut back some and no one else knows I still have one or two a day. Oh—there's the turn...*It feels better in my mouth than it does bloating my stomach after I downed the extreme size. I was able to find a trash in a retail store parking lot to dump the cup a couple miles up the road so it is nearly like it didn't happen. Except for the physical results and, of course, the shame that I am harboring by sneaking around. Now both my body and self-esteem are hurting. *I really need to stop doing that. Why do I do that?*

Have you ever experienced one of these stories in your own life? My guess is that we all have in one form or another. What does it take to get past these types of situations? How do we develop mental stamina so that it doesn't feel like such a wrestling match? I want to enjoy my life, my food, and my time with others without all these voices arguing in my head. Stop. Just make it stop.

Do you agree? Well, read on through this and I know that you will feel armed with a better understanding of what is going on in your head.

CHAPTER FIVE

Illuminate The Path

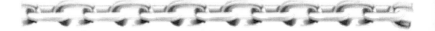

Chains are durable and cannot simply be shattered. You must use the right tools to break free. There are three specific tools that we can use to escape the chains that we accept as a result of our decisions. This is not intended to be a comprehensive list, but it does provide a sense of how we can actually take real steps towards the life that looks more like what we dream of. But before we can loosen the chains, we must first acknowledge the momentary choices we make that thwart our dreams.

Advanced Choice

I decided I was not going to do drugs when I was little. I don't actually even remember the date, time, or my age when I made that decision. I do know that it was not made in the heat or pressure of the moment. I decided *before* I was ever in a position to make a bad choice. I knew that these substances were not going to be a part of my future by specific choice—advanced choice.

Advanced choice is powerful and important because it allows us to make decisions with only a fraction of the willpower that it requires in the moment. If we could predetermine each of our situations and circumstances then we could decide in advance how to react. There are many examples in life where we really should take this approach, but unfortunately this is not a universally available tool to depend on because we simply cannot anticipate everything we will face.

Take this opportunity to think of something challenging that you will face in the next 24 hours and decide how you will positively react. Do it now. Practice and see that what I am saying is true. When you decided in advance, it makes the moments of pressure easier to handle. You have already informed yourself how you are going to respond. That may be very different than how you have responded in the past.

Determination

I told my mom when I was four years old that I wanted to drive racecars. For all of my life that I can remember, I have been enamored by the love of the sport of racing. My heart yearns for competition and the pursuit of excellence in what I do. In my early teens I dreamed of being an engineer for a big company such as General Motors.

These dreams required the use of advanced choice and determination to make them reality. When establishing vision, you have to actually visualize where it is that you want to be. In so doing, you build passion that fuels determination. Without determination, we cannot accomplish any of our goals.

So, we all have dreams. To see those dreams thrive, we need to apply some good ole fashion determination. But, sometimes determination can be fleeting so we need some horsepower behind it. I find that if I write out my dreams or draw pictures of them or even make a model to look at then this process and the mental clarity that comes along with it helps provide the strength that my determination needs to stay alive.

Goals are dreams in writing which create a vision. It is what you want to happen. As soon as you complete these wonderful writings, you will begin to face challenges. Thankfully, you can share your goals with others and in exchange you will get encouragement, if you share it with the right people! We all know that the challenges are much more common than the encouragement. Determination is really a form of self-encouragement.

A strategy to success is to apply copious amounts of determination! That makes it sound a bit easier than it may seem to you. What I have found is that determination in anything is easier if we are consistent in all of our commitments. Giving up is a bad habit. If we give up in the minor commitments in our lives then we will be more prone to giving up on the big commitments. Therefore, don't volunteer for things that you do not intend to fully complete. Take more time, if needed, to consider all of your commitments because the results of each will build or destroy your propensity to complete tasks consistently. Make a habit of intentional commitment for the next month, noting on your calendar the end date to see how you are doing.

It all distills down to the fact that determination is a habit. It is the result of a person who does what he vows and completes what he commits to consistently. In my view, this is the most important key to effectively applying determination. We must make a habit of it.

It's Just Meant To Be

How much control do we really have over our life, results, choices, and circumstances? I don't know the answer to that question but the thought makes me consider the alternatives.

We can't be robots because that would just ruin everything that we know and believe. I do not believe that God made us to be robots. Why would we need Jesus and His grace if we were unable to make mistakes? Instead, I believe that we need Him because we have free will and are able to chart our own course in life.

What if there was something else in control that was actually within our reach but we just didn't realize it? Stay with me here. I have thought about this for years and believe there are nuggets of truth here that will help us get free of our food chains.

I believe we have a comprehensive worldview in life that determines how we make decisions. What causes you to choose right or left in a situation when it doesn't matter? Why do you choose a certain dish on a menu, song on the radio, side of the bed, outfit, reaction, drink, or activity? Some of these things you can attribute to favorites, habits, or choices but is there more to it than that?

Why do you believe that a certain outfit makes you look better when compared to another? You may not consciously consider that when deciding what to wear but that perception will have its impact in your decision. What if you think a certain type of food will provider better health benefits (regardless of the truth)? That knowledge will impact your decisions.

Bigger picture. What if you believe certain things about yourself, who you are and whose you are? What if that belief is not as good as it really should be? For example, what if you don't believe you deserve to live well, to win, to be attractive, and to succeed wildly?

So, does our belief system impact our moment-by-moment choices? Or do those choices end up subject to our circumstances in the moment? I believe the former, that our belief system drives our lives by directing our decisions with every choice we make. Let me explain how.

Each time we face a decision, we toss the available information over the wall to our sub-conscience to get direction on how we should respond. Think I am crazy? Analyze your decisions these next few days. You will find that you are not actually in control of how you react. Well, not directly. What is in control is your system of belief? What you believe about your life and your circumstances is more important than the reality of the situation. You will make decisions in every situation that supports what you believe.

The obvious line of thinking must now shift to how we adjust our belief system so that we can make choices that are more in line with what it is that we really want to see happen. I have studied this in my own life for years and the common problem is that what I want to believe is not actually what I truly believe. Our belief system is really our foundation. If our belief system is bent a certain way then that is how our decisions will be skewed.

It takes a lot of time and patience to change the belief system. First, you have to realize that there is incongruence between what you believe and what you want to believe. Self-reflection and others' input is necessary to see these deep-rooted beliefs that are hindering the life you hope to live. Change the false belief and you will see the results begin to transform on their own.

As I look at this, I am leading you to think about your circumstances and to question how much of your passions played a role in guiding you in making daily choices. Are there other factors that impact these choices? Could some of these actually be putting us in chains that we don't even see? Are we in a form of voluntary prison due to our choices? If yes, then what is causing us to continue making choices that perpetuate our live in chains?

CHAPTER SIX

Voluntarily In Chains

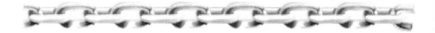

The importance of actively looking into the future is well established. Unfortunately, nearly everything in our culture today is assisting us in avoiding thinking about our future. Everything we need is at our fingertips at nearly every moment of the day. Every nook and cranny of our time is filled so full that we don't even have time to think about the future, even if it did interest us. When we do have free time we struggle to know what to do with ourselves. We think that it is a waste of time to sit and think about deep thoughts. We have become a culture of zombies.

How could life improve if we did establish some form of clarity about the future? What if we spent a few minutes each daydreaming about the future? Could we come up with a few new ideas each week? Could we carry these into the days ahead and use them to build a long-term vision for our ideal lives? What if on those nights when we can't seem to sleep, we replaced mindless TV with scribbling down ideas and dreams? What if we kept an ongoing note on our mobile device to capture ideas as they came to us? What if we brainstormed ideas with our friends and family to spark something? Would any of that have an effect on whom we become and what we accomplish? Furthermore, would it have an effect on our motivation to succeed – to win?

Let's establish some definitions of common forms of envisioning the future.

Vision: A vision is the effect of us considering our future and establishing a portrait of what we think will happen. A vision can be in our minds or it can be written or drawn out as a picture or a story.

Mission: A mission is a list of action items that are established after examining a well-documented vision. Once you understand your vision then you can use that as a goal and work back from there to establish a mission.

Goals: Goals are stated (personal or public) destinations that you plan to reach. The size of the destination may be small, even in the form of tiny little steps, or could be much a larger accomplishment. To qualify as a goal, your destination must have a clearly articulated vision and missional steps to accomplish the vision.

Desires, Dreams & Dreaming: Dreams are plentiful and often only a minority of our dreams actually graduate into mission steps. Dreams are important as they often assist in painting the portrait of our overall vision. They also act as guideposts as we grow and mature, often becoming more selfless in our understanding of our life, vision, and resulting mission. Dreaming is fun and should be encouraged. Dreams should be shared openly and recipients should practice listening with excitement, encouragement, and enjoyment.

A downfall of dreams in our society is that we tend to dream when we are young and we have lots of time. We organize all those dreams to neatly fit into one of the many shoeboxes we acquire in our childhood. As we grow up we are taught to stop dreaming, as it is perceived to be childish. So we place our dreams into our shoebox and store them at our parents' while we go off to college to "do the right thing." We get caught up in the crowd of real thinkers during those years. When we return to start paying off our college loans, we retrieve our stuff from our parents' and move it to our new home. Of course we are secretly excited to grab our shoebox of dreams and we carefully place it on the mantle above our fireplace. Over time, we get more comfortable with our dreams just being about who we were when we were children or who we once hoped we would be. We may get courageous and occasionally share the contents of our box with our friends. But eventually we accept that they are never going to be something that defines reality for our lives. There they sit however until we get married, move, or when we finally cross one of the many bridges in life where we decide to leave our dreams behind forever.

The truth is that we are made to dream. We dream when we sleep and we dream when we are awake. Our dreams drive our deepest desires and motivations. Our dreams cause us to take on projects that will stretch us. Our dreams take us places we would never otherwise go. Our dreams open up opportunities for us to meet people who help us achieve the impossible. Our dreams are the things that make up our vision for what our lives will become. Our dreams are the foundation to our legacy.

Because we do not take the time to use these future-shaping tools, our lives become the result of our momentary choices. In so doing, we submit to the chains and shackles of this world. We trade what could be with whatever happens. We choose to be chained down by the expectations of this world instead of charting our own course as driven by our vision.

Without vision, momentary desires become what we live for. People choose to live for sex, money, control, influence, status, all manner of vices, and, of course, the next meal.

Think about it: what will excite you most in the next few days? I guarantee that it includes at least one of your personal vices (even if you don't recognize it yet), and it likely includes food.

When I have tested myself of these things, I have found myself feeling unstable, uncomfortable, an—ironically—even bored.

Here is an example of how you can test yourself in this area. Plan to attend a gathering for a greater purpose other than food or service. It can be a social event, family gathering, or even a business adventure. Attend the event after a light, healthy snack (piece of fruit, fresh smoothie, etc.).

For me, it became abundantly clear that I didn't care nearly enough about people and the time that I had to simply be with them, to learn about their interests, desires, and pains. I wanted the food! I was there for the food! I was astounded when this was confirmed time after time. If I didn't value people and time with them, then what good could I be to anyone—other than myself? Doing these tests kicked off a big change in my thinking. I realized how much I worshiped food and I realize that I did not desire to know and love people nearly as much as I should—and, in truth, how much I really wanted to. Coming to this place was the starting point for change in my mind.

Going through these experiences really helped me to see that my motivations were foul. I was allowing the momentary to take over control that my vision should have been dictating. If I was truly living for my vision (in this case, serving people) then my actions would be driven from my mission and I would be actively pursuing my goals. In turn I would be preparing myself for long-term success.

The great challenge with this is all the moments for seemingly instantaneously-satisfying actions. Our lives are filled with opportunities for immediate pleasure. Many of the options may certainly be fun or pleasurable, but nearly all of them will also move us slightly away from our vision. I cannot think of a more appropriate example aside from food and our diet. Thanks to all manner of chemical additives, our food does often taste amazing. A bite here and a meal there; before we know it we have eaten our way into a few extra sizes and worse – a very unhealthy state overall. This leads to at least slight depression and ends up impacting the overall balance in our thinking. It also builds and develops deep-rooted habits that tend to keep us on the same path.

My desire is that we would dream big, cast vision, understand our mission, and write down our goals. In so doing, we will move closer to avoiding the moment-by-moment lies that keep us from experiencing the great rewards of actualizing our vision!

What are you dreaming about today? What did you dream about years ago that has affected who you are and where you ended up today? Can you list dreams that you had long ago that simply went unanswered? You know, the ones that just seemed impossible so they stayed hung on the walls of your mind like artwork and never became reality?

Even thought they went unanswered, those dreams still contributed to shaping who you are today.

What are you dreaming about today and how are you actively enabling that to shape tomorrow? If you are not sure then you are likely living in the chains that are formed when you serve the momentary idols that promise to make us happy but never actually deliver. This is the day when all that is going to change for you. It is time to break the chains and shackles that are holding you from achieving your dreams.

When we live like this, we avoid the chains and shackles that are stamped with our name on them along the path of our lives. It is time to get free!

CHAPTER SEVEN

Vision Is Long Term

How many times have you heard stories of a couple struggling in their marriage who head off to a weekend seminar and come back revitalized, possibly even pregnant? Maybe this example isn't too distant for you. It certainly is a popular one, and on the surface it seems like a very good result. Likely in some cases, the value that comes from such a weekend, or maybe pieces of it, contributes to an overall end result that is better than where they were before. Maybe it is a series of these seminars that builds up to a crescendo where something just clicks and he (or she) finally gets it.

As you read this, know that I am all for continuing education. In fact, I made a point of including a chapter on that very subject in this book. Also, I am not saying that we should avoid these weekend seminars and other types of on-going education. It's quite the opposite, in fact. If you take a look at my wife's and my schedule, we are proving it in our own lives.

For some of us however, we do need to adjust our perspective on why and how we go about these opportunities. More often than not the result is something like the following: A couple finds themselves at a point in their relationship a few months after the wedding when the bliss and newness of the marriage wears off. Now they have a chance to live together and they realize how annoying they each are. She snores at night and for some reason doesn't always look as put-together as she did on their dates. He seems a bit lazy and always seems to be chasing some prize—other than her. After all, she is won already, right? They have some friends who mention they are attending a seminar in a couple weeks, so this couple signs up as well.

The seminar comes and the education is amazing. The result is wonderful, and they actually feel higher after the weekend than they did on their honeymoon. What a difference some focus can make! They float in the clouds for a few days until signs of the same patterns that dragged them down previously begin to become apparent once again.

I call the weekend seminar "the spike" and the ensuing months "the slide." Not too many months later they find themselves in about the same place, if not a little lower, than they felt before. Now they have the burden of realizing that the seminar was a bit of a hot shot at best and that there are still severe problems. They insist it must have been the wrong seminar, so they sign up for another weekend seminar. Off they go successfully training themselves to live the spike and slide instead of actually growing.

This is not an uncommon scenario in our culture. What is the problem? Clearly that isn't the point of this book so let me give you the short version: apathy, laziness, lack of trust in God, false idols, desires that become expectations, men who simply don't understand themselves (seriously, woman are not the confusing ones), pride, arrogance, sin, folly, Satan, mistakes, false paradigms, and inaccurate world views.

The point of this section is that this couple, as well as anyone trying to lose weight, who succeeds in something such as overcoming an illness or stopping a habit, will face similar mental challenges as they adventure along. How will they respond to these challenges? How will this couple respond after seventeen weekend seminars with the same spike-and-slide results? Are they willing to face the facts of their situation? Are they over-optimistic about their circumstances? Will they give up?

Admiral Jim Stockdale served in the United States Navy during the Vietnam War. He was a prisoner-of-war, was tortured and beaten without the slightest hope of being released. Stockdale secretly led a group of prisoners through a mental journey that lasted him eight years.

According to the account in Jim Collins' best-selling book, *Good to Great*, the Admiral indicated that the optimistic didn't survive. Those who set false targets, such as being released by Christmas, would end up dying of a broken heart. Those who simply faced the fact that they did not have a date for release, but yet were somehow able to continue to believe they would be set free, were the survivors.

Collins accurately defines the relationship between endurance and success, where people's success is inextricably tied to how well they persevered through repeated failure in personal goals, all the while balancing the reality of personal limitations. Collins calls this "The Stockdale Paradox," where we are challenged to "retain faith that we will prevail in the end, regardless of the difficulties." At the same time, we are to "confront the most brutal facts of our current reality, whatever they might be."

So, it seems that successful people are those who can maintain a stoic focus on the goal while, at the same time, honestly recognizing their circumstances and abilities. This does not mean that just because I might be three laps down with a mediocre racecar that I can't somehow come back to win the race. It simply means I need to stay focused on winning while at the same time understanding my situation. In a racing situation, this focus enables a team to make decisions they may not otherwise make, in order to earn back laps they otherwise would not have gained.

So what does all of this have to do with diet and lifestyle? The lesson here is to choose: Do you want to make a big change, only to slide back to where you are now—or worse? Or, do you want to invest heavily in education, make small changes, and maintain a stoic focus on where you want to be years from now? Clearly, these are opposite directions and the results are going to be substantially different as well. It is the difference between a marriage and a date. Casually dating a healthy lifestyle isn't going to get you the results you want. Committed marriage, with a vision for what can be, presents your best chance for success.

Food impacts every one of us. It was even the tool Satan used to entrap Adam and Eve, and I believe he continues to use it today to taunt us and to lead us astray. A friend of mine recently helped me to see this more clearly. He said that the love of food is the only false idol you can't just knock down and walk away from. A person can choose to not partake in gambling, an addiction, laziness, or sexual sin because they are not vital to survival. In so doing, they are saying that they choose God, the real Deity, over their false idol. But what about the sin of gluttony (the excessive love of food)? We still need the nourishment that comes from the food, so we need to continue to eat. We can't just kick it to the curb like the bottle. It is likely for this reason that it is very difficult for people to openly see the reality of their relationship to their food.

For those of you who do finally achieve a glimpse of the mastering control that your food has on you, you can successfully begin to apply the principals of the Stockdale Paradox successfully. You will begin to see the truth about your situation and the control that has been yielded to food. You will recognize the impact that your food and lifestyle choices have on your existence. From there, you can begin to build hope that you will be able to achieve success in using food for fuel, and refocusing your life on eating to live rather than living to eat. Realizations like this are sobering and they remind me of sayings like "ignorance is bliss." Hopefully I have not ruined your bliss. Well, maybe I do hope that I have. I believe the challenges we face after bliss are purposed to take us to a greater joy.

So, you may ask, when will it start to feel as good? Based on what we learned about the Stockdale Paradox, the answer to that is very likely going to be different for every person. If I told you so many days, weeks, or even years, then that would be setting you up like one of Stockdale's over-optimists. Not only that, but your situation is uniquely yours and by that very nature has a unique set of circumstances. What I will promise you is that the path does get sweet, and there are innumerable treasures in plain sight along the way that are left for you to enjoy.

CHAPTER EIGHT

Taking Ownership

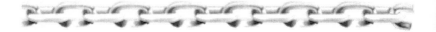

Excuses pervade our lives and prevent us from achieving most of what we actually want and what is possible. The problem is that it is difficult for us to see when we are making excuses for ourselves and sometimes for those close to us.

Think about the thing that you wish you could stop doing. Maybe it is eating sugary stuff you know isn't good for you. Or the big meaty hot dogs loaded with sauerkraut and mustard. Could be that coffee, soda, or energy drink. Some would like to drop a smoking habit. Others are struggling with lying, cheating, or sneaking. Some people just talk too much and they know it but can't seem to stop.

Wouldn't it be nice if you could just wake up and be free of the bondage that this thing has over you? If you're disagreeing with me that such things have control over you then just stop for three weeks and see if you agree.

You may disagree that this activity is controlling you. Maybe it isn't. Maybe the result that it gives is literally the sorry version of your potential. Or, maybe you don't believe that the negative effects that are proven to come from repeated retreat to this thing will actually affect you. Or, maybe you just refuse to believe that the literature and research about the thing is actually true. Or, even more frightening, maybe you don't have a vision for your life that is bigger than the results you are getting by clinging to your vice day after day.

Many people go down this path and the words that surface are addiction, personality, or habit. It could very well be a habit that you have made. Key word is you. *You* choose the habit and *you* can choose a new one. If you lean on the idea that this is a trap of your personality then you could be right—to an extent. That is the easy excuse because you are suggesting that your parents brought you up a certain way so it is really their fault. That works for a while until you have kids and they start saying such things until you gently remind them that they have their own brain and willpower. Don't blame it on your parents. Take ownership of your habits.

The addiction word is a tougher one. This is where I will likely irritate you. But, stick with me here because I have studied this in my only life and in the lives of others for years and know what I am about to tell you is true.

Your addictions are your chosen vices. Yes, you choose your addictions. And, as you would expect, I know that you can un-choose them.

You were born with the choice to walk a different path. You are not destined for the negative results of living through momentary pleasure.

No matter how much control you have turned over to your vice(s), you can take it back. And, it is very likely that you can completely reverse the results that you accrued over time. You cannot make up for the dreary days that you have experienced thus far but that should certainly motivate you to change.

At the end, there is a truth that is the same for each of us. We are the only ones who are going to truly affect change in our own lives. The day we each realize that we accepted the chains we live in, the sooner we will begin to move into a place of peace, realizing that we are equally as able to live our dreams.

It is yet another example of us giving up great long-term results to feel better or to experience some sort of satisfaction in the moment. The truth is that the momentary pleasure comes of a great cost – the cost of our dreams.

CHAPTER NINE

Rejected for Dead

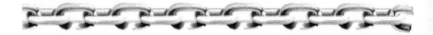

It has not been all roses since my diagnosis. It has been great, but we have also made some mistakes and faced some challenges. The biggest one for me was dehydration the first couple of years.

It took me several years to shift my diet to 80% or more raw foods. During that time, and probably years before, I had been dehydrating myself. On one occasion, I was scheduled for a speaking engagement about an hour from our home and was suddenly feeling terrible. I was tired, weak, had a headache, and was very thirsty. I had only two hours before I was supposed to be on stage. We recognized dehydration and I quickly started drinking water. After several glasses and about 20 minutes I felt able to speak again. The hydration was key because the presentation was on an outdoor stage in direct sunlight.

I eat primarily raw foods now, so hydration is not an issue with me any longer, but it is really important to find a healthy balance in your hydration. Outside of my workouts, I rarely drink water. This is only possible because I consume considerable water through my raw food consumption.

Deadly Toxins

During the first two years, we ate a lot of what we called "transitional foods." These were generally foods that were vegan (100% free of animal products, including dairy), but cooked. A good example is the "Vegan" taco served at a local Mexican food bar. I ate there regularly during those first couple of years. Remember, I mentioned earlier that I started using my body as my barometer for determining what food made my body feel good. After a while I started to notice I didn't feel well after eating the vegan burrito. At first I thought it was because of the generous portion, but research revealed the problem was actually chemicals in my food—specifically monosodium glutamate (MSG). This particular company, like many fast food establishments, does not actually cook any of their food in the restaurant. It is processed in a huge food factory.

The Only Rule for Food Manufacturing:

Rule#1: It must be profitable while not causing immediate death.

Summary: If immediate death can be avoided then put all remaining emphasis on product profitability.

Yes, this may be a bit tongue-in-cheek—but it still rings true. Is it just me, or does the thought of eating a lunch that was made in a factory seem wrong? Not the lunch room of a factory, but a factory that is specifically built to process and create food for us. My background is in manufacturing engineering, so thinking about factories and building things is not unusual for me. Have you ever considered where your food was made? There is a show on a cable network called "How It's Made" that often shows some of these food factory settings. One episode I watched recently with my kids showed how hot dogs were made. The audible response from them was comical and wonderful at the same time!

They showed a very large stainless steel mixing bowl of sorts. It was literally about the size of a small dump truck. That wasn't so bad, but watching them pour huge lumps of animal parts and pieces jammed together with fat and dripping with blood grossed out my kids.

The bowl was, of course, some sort of mixing machine. This was the initial stage of combining the proper ingredients to make the desired type of hot dogs. The mix was then fed into a grinding machine, which eliminated any tiny animal body parts from surviving intact. Next, they showed how they stretch out the cow guts (intestinal sleeve-like pieces) to create the outer casing that will hold the mix together while it cooks. This was the fun part for the kids, because the goop shot out of the end of a machine into the sleeve-like intestines at a rate of about 1000 dogs per minute. After that, the dogs were cooked, the sleeve was sliced off, and the cooked hot dog-shaped slop headed to the packaging area. They also showed a similar mix used to fill up bread-shaped pans before cooking. These loaves were used for sliced sandwich meat.

I once drew this diagram. The box represents what we choose to label as food, while the small circle represents what actually is nourishing food—or, *real* food.

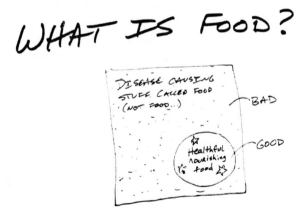

The point is, we tend to feel comfortable eating stuff that is packaged in an appealing way by a worker in a factory. Does anything seem wrong with this? One of the books and movies I recommend is *Fast Food Nation*. In it you will learn about the mechanical and business aspects of food manufacturing. If a company's primary purpose is profitability, then how much concern are they really going to take in ensuring that the food they create is good for you? Furthermore, if God created all the food we need in nature, then are we not playing god by attempting to modify or create new food?

Food made in a factory is filled with chemicals to make it taste good after all the life is cooked out of it. It arrives in the restaurants in big plastic bags and is either microwaved or steamed to temperature. This food comes off the assembly line flavorless because cooking removes the majority of the flavor. Flavor additives are then added back into the food during and after cooking.

As an experiment, I decided to investigate the ingredients in a can of Campbell's Cream of Mushroom soup. I did a bit of research online and quickly realized that they do not share their ingredients online. I even emailed their customer support and was told I needed to visit a store and actually look at the label.

Give me a break. They can chant all they want about secret, company-owned recipes, but it is a bunch of marketing bunk. A six-year-old with a well-stocked kitchen and a little help could replicate and possibly even improve upon any of their products in a couple hours. They are not hiding anything other than the fact that they are using massive amounts of excitotoxins in their food. Excitotoxins began with the additive called monosodium glutamate, or MSG. Because MSG has to be listed on the ingredients list when it is included within a manufactured food, it is now sold under more than one hundred different disguised names such as hydrolyzed protein, sodium caseinate, yeast extract, textured protein and many others. Additionally L-cysteine, aspartate, and aspartame are excitotoxins that are not required by the FDA to be shown on food labeling. As if that wasn't bad enough, names like natural flavoring, bouillon, seasoning, malt extract, spices, carrageenan, enzymes, and many more are often hiding places for manufacturers to include excitotoxins in the foods they produce. In other words, some food manufacturers want to make it as difficult as possible for people to know all ingredients, regardless of the dangers that they know they pose to the consumer.

So what is the big deal with an excitotoxin and why should we be so concerned about them? According to Dr. Russell L. Blaylock in his book, *Excitotoxins*, these are a group of excitatory amino acids that can cause sensitive neurons to die. Some of these compounds are found in nature and some are created artificially, such as kainate. When a neuron is exposed to a massive dose of MSG, the cell immediately begins to swell and dies within one hour. When a lower dose of MSG is used, nothing appears to happen immediately, but after the second hour the neuron suddenly undergoes rapid death.

I had the displeasure of experiencing two very unfortunate incidents of chemical poisoning, and both occurred just after eating at Mexican restaurants. One was after a meal at one of the locations of a fast, casual Mexican food chain in Seattle and the other was just after a meal at a local Mexican restaurant in Eagle, Idaho. Both experiences turned out to be two of the most uncomfortable, painful situations I can remember and brought me closer to death than the cancer did. During a family vacation, we had to extend our time at a lake in McCall, Idaho, because I was in bed for about thirty-six hours, and I wasn't sure if I was going to live. I couldn't eat anything and all I could drink was water. I was chemically poisoned and in a lot of pain. I could not sleep for more than an hour or two at a time and I just hurt all over. Chemical poisoning is very different than congestion or a virus or similar types of illnesses. It comes quickly, significantly hurts, has to be flushed out, and then leaves rather swiftly. After a couple of days of struggling in pain, drinking water, and lying in bed, it finally passed and I returned to feeling fine. The reaction to a meal at the local fast, casual Mexican restaurant was less severe.

To be clear, our family does enjoy eating at certain Mexican food restaurants. We often get a variation of a veggie fajita dish with tortilla wraps or served over a bed of greens. We are just super careful to verify that the restaurant does not use any excitotoxins such as MSG.

Rejection

During the period of weeks and months after my cancer diagnosis, I remember thinking I should get a t-shirt saying, "Why are you treating me like I am going to die soon?" It was amazing how people wrote me off. There is something about having a terminal illness that makes others want to disassociate themselves from you. Fortunately, I am married to my wonderful wife, Nikki, and she mitigated the hurt from such callous responses (so I never got the t-shirt). However, I talked with other survivors and this does seem to be a common response from the people around them. I can remember when I associated "cancer" with "death" almost as directly as I associated "fast" with "racing!" When I hear of someone with a diagnosis of cancer now, I get excited because I realize there is a cure. People who receive a cancer diagnosis are most likely going to have the motivation necessary to make some serious changes.

Yes, it is exciting…when they listen to truth.

As I talk with others who have had a terminal or near-terminal diagnosis, I find we all share a common experience in the way we felt about the human reaction to impending death. The initial reaction is shock. Some people desire to help, but most seek the answer to the inevitable question, *"why?"* Romans 12:2 indicates that if we want to know the will of God for our lives through testing and approval, then we must first be transformed. How? By the renewal of our minds. *"Do not be conformed to this world, but be transformed by the renewal of your mind, that by testing you may discern what is the will of God, what is good and acceptable and perfect."* (ESV)

Well, I certainly want to know God's will for my life, so how do I renew my mind? I mention this Scripture here not because I intend to fully answer the question of how we change, but because I want to demonstrate that it's futile to ask the "why" question of God every time things don't go as we plan. We are much better served by getting to know His plan for us in His great story.

Other cancer survivors recount how family, friends, and coworkers drift away over time. The relationships begin to die because the people think the person is facing certain death. It is easier for them to create some physical separation so when the day comes that they hear our life has ended, the pain will be somewhat mitigated.

For those like me who live through the diagnosis, the more human reaction becomes bizarre. People act as if nothing ever happened. I think this took about five years for me. With some people, it is still uncomfortable when we see each other. I know you are probably thinking, *Isn't that what you want, for people to treat you normally?* Well, yes and no. I want people to treat me normally just as all of us do, but I also want people to recognize that God did a miracle through me, and He wants to do one through you as well.

Maybe you don't have cancer or a severe physical problem at all. Maybe He wants to heal you in your marriage or your relationship with your family. It could be that He wants to work a miracle through mistakes you have made in your past that still hold you back today. The point is He wants the best for us, and it is ridiculous for us to look into the face of a beautiful scene, created by God, and ignore His desires to work in all of us. All we need to do is be willing to participate in actively seeking Him to learn what our part in the process.

Allergies

You can check with my mom, but I was the allergy prince as a kid. My eyes would swell shut if someone even mentioned the season of spring! I didn't get sick regularly, but I had my fair share of viral illnesses.

In the years I have been doing this, I would estimate my allergy issues are over 90 percent better and often non-existent. Sometimes I may need to refine my diet, or I may need to eliminate a chemical or issue that is bothering my body. For instance, I got pink eye in 2006, which was sort of uncomfortable but looked much worse than it felt. I was told it was a virus and would be tough to avoid regardless of my health. I didn't visit the doctor for it and only took natural oils recommended by a friend. It was pretty amazing how quickly it passed. The oils, for reference, were oregano and rosemary. Don't ask me how they worked, but I can tell you that there is more about essential oils that I need to learn in the coming years.

We need to openly consider alternative theories about allergies because we can easily be deceived by the modern philosophy. I began to learn about this a few years ago when someone told me that they were allergic to a food that I felt, by design, there should be no allergy. The food was spinach, but that doesn't really matter because I have heard people say this about all different types of food. Nuts and grains tend to be the most common, and there may actually be some validity to their claims with these because most nuts and grains are processed. So, the question is, are we allergic to the food item, or to the processing, including possible added substances? Even with produce, could it be that we are actually allergic to the chemicals that are used to speed the growth, size and perfection of the produce? These questions may help us isolate the root cause and eliminate allergies in the future.

Simply identifying the properties of the food or substance would be relatively simple. If we are allergic to spinach then we simply avoid spinach or maybe we look at what spinach is made up of to try to determine if there is some property of the spinach that is the actual culprit. Again, I believe this is the obvious response but it ignores the real issue. Our allergic reaction to many substances must be a symptom of a different problem.

An allergic reaction is defined as an over-reaction of our self-healing system, our immune defenses. For some reason, our internal army has been summoned to fight an enemy, but in some cases, our protective army over-reacts against what should be considered harmless or possibly even helpful. It is important to recognize that this immune reaction is natural and necessary function of our overall immune system but at times it explodes into an over-reaction.

Let me use an example. You walk out your front door and water drips on your head. The ground is wet and you know it's been raining. You happen to have had an elaborate gutter system installed on your house that is supposed to catch the water from the roof and divert it to downspouts and an alternate drainage system. You look at the gutters and assume they've failed to do their job. You try caulking the joints but still water is dripping on your head. You try putting diverters on the roof to funnel the water a different direction, but still water is dripping on your head. In all of your efforts to fix the gutters you failed to realize that gutters only capture some of the problem. Dripping gutters are a sign (symptom) that it is raining. The fact that it is raining is the source of the problem.

Likewise, we have created unpredictable environments within our bodies because of the toxins we ingest with eating and breathing. We can't simply say we are allergic to this or that without a deeper consideration of the environment we have created in our bodies by our lifestyle choices. This is especially true if the things we are claiming to be allergic to are natural foods made by our Designer. If you get a headache after eating an orange or a rash after eating broccoli, then clearly there is another problem. That problem is not the orange or the broccoli. If you experience an allergic reaction after consuming something that should be nutritional and beneficial then there is a deeper problem inside the body, not inside the healthy food.

I have spoken with several Chron's Disease sufferers tell me that they were told to avoid all greens due to some issues that cause flare-ups within their digestive systems. What they are actually being told is to avoid fiber because the fiber is abrasive to the digestive system. This abrasiveness is irritating and uncomfortable to an already compromised system. This scenario represents the very same thing I am saying about allergies. The very thing that all of us need as a primary piece of our diet is raw, leafy, dark greens. In the case of a Crohn's patient, they may need to juice these and attempt to avoid fiber as much as possible until they improve the internal condition. For allergies, we need to consider the overall health of our system, make changes to improve deficiencies, and not get distracted along the way because what we know to be true doesn't seem to be working.

Be skeptical of direct cause-and-effect lines drawn between any food and any allergic reaction. Realize that other factors inside your body contribute to the allergic reaction just as much, if not more, than what you actually ate. If I were allergic to some natural food that God clearly designed for us to enjoy, then I would look at the rest of my diet and overall toxic load (past and present) to try to determine what may be contributing to this reaction. I would make some changes and test again until the allergy symptoms disappeared. In other words, test for allergies and then change the condition in your body until the symptoms disappear.

There are some things that are not designed to eat and will kill us instantly. Other things were clearly designed for us to ingest for our nourishment and benefit. It is interesting that we are smart enough to avoid the things that will kill us instantly, yet we choose to accept the consumption of those things that cause slow death.

My family generally lives free of allergies and sicknesses. We never have to clean out our noses or sinuses in the shower like I can remember doing in the past. I believe this pattern of health enables our family to live with less stress, fatigue and uncontrolled emotions. In other words, because of our lifestyle choices, life is just easier in our home than in many homes. We do have a wonderful family and an incredibly fun family life. This is in part possible due to our healthy diet choices.

CHAPTER TEN

Cause of Dis-ease

Heart disease, cancer, diabetes, osteoporosis, autoimmune issues, obesity, Crohn's Disease, and *fill-in-the-blank* are all caused by the same thing. Shocked? I get it. I was too when I learned this truth. Disease is caused by cellular disorders. Those cellular disorders simply manifest themselves in different ways within our bodies. Many of the diseases are, by name, merely a memorial for the doctor or scientist that identified and named it.

Lets look at cancer as an example. Cancer can show up in all sorts of parts of the body right? We hear of people getting brain cancer or stomach cancer or prostate, liver, skin, breast cancer. How can the same disease show up in so many different places? Cancer is a mutation of cells somewhere in your body that causes cells to grow in an abnormal way. The cells are mutated yet our body does not recognize them as foreign and allows them to continue to replicate, grow, feed off of and starve the surrounding tissue. The issue with cancer begins at the cellular level. Though cells have gone awry, the immune system is too weakened to be able to recognize the problem. It is important to note that cancer commonly exists in all of our bodies. A healthy immune system understands and is built to combat this. So, the issue is not actually a war on cancer as much as it should be a battle to strengthen our immune system.

Lets now look at diabetes, especially type 2 diabetes. This is a softball because everyone knows diabetes is a chosen disease, right? Well, not everyone I talk to. They act like it is something to suffer under forever. Many rebuff the thought that nearly all symptoms of diabetes could be completely gone within three weeks if they simply changed their diet. Enough ranting, diabetes is a cellular-level disease. The pancreas is over-exerted to the point where they simply can't produce at the level necessary. Why is it overworked? Because of diet. The pancreas was simply not designed to function at such a high level, which leads to exhaustion. I have even heard of promising stories of children suffering from type 1 diabetes where it can be improved and even reversed with diet and lifestyle alignment.

What about something like osteoporosis? How is this a problem at the cellular level? Ironically, osteoporosis is closely tied to diabetes because it is a fully diet-attributed disease. Osteoporosis is chosen through our diet. No amount of artificial calcium supplementation can make up for what we are doing to our bodies by allowing a poor diet made up of acidic foods that erode calcium from our bones. When we eat these acid-forming foods, our body is forced to scavenge a neutralizer to try to control the results of the acid, ultimately bone calcium. Thus, the more acid we consume, the less dense our bones become. Ironically (or not), some of the worst acid-forming foods contain artificial calcium supplementation which doesn't actually make up for the damage it causes.

What causes disease?

Toxins cause diseases. You can also look at it as a toxic load in excess of our physical ability to overcome. I have explained this in the past as a balance scale. If the toxins are stacked up on the left, then we need to pile the same amount of nutrition, or immunity building blocks, on the right. It really is that simple. Overcome the toxic load and you will completely avoid physical ailments.

Toxins can be in our food but can also come from other sources. The air we breathe, clothes we wear, and people we make contact with can all contribute to our toxic load. It can even come from stress. This can lead to actual physical toxicity of our own making and cause physical or physiological breakdown.

How is disease cured?

There are only two ways your body can be cured and neither one is a pill. There is no pill that has ever cured anything and suggesting that it does is pure insanity. Pills mask symptoms, which is why we continue to take them. The issue or disease is not cured—it is hidden by the work of the pill. If it is possible, would it not be better to cure the problem rather than mask the symptoms?

The first method to being cured is the most common method by far. This is healing that takes place due to our built-in self-healing mechanisms. It is our responsibility to nourish our bodies in such a way that we enable these internal functions to operate properly. The second method for curing disease is much less commonly experienced—it purely by the grace of God working in us. It is an absolute possibility, but to our knowledge, rarely enacted—at least not how we expect.

Am I cursed because of my genes?

No. You may have some stronger predispositions towards a certain disease or ailment, but you are not cursed or destined to die of what ails your parents, grandparents, cousins, or other family members. Your biggest family risk factor is actually in how much your daily habits reflect theirs. In other words, the fact that you mimic the same behavior as your parents is more powerful than the fact that you got your genes from them. Stop doing the bad things that they do and you will experience different results.

Another factor to consider when looking at your family history is what I call 'generational degeneration.' With each passing generation our toxic environment there is a compounding of physical brokenness. Someone who is unhealthy is going to pass on not only their unhealthy habits but also their disease proclivities. This is exacerbated by the rapid decline in overall food quality in recent generations. What this looks like in practice is that people are getting diagnosed at younger ages and showing signs of general ailing sooner than previous generations. This plays out until we begin to experience infertility which in many cases is simply a physical response from the body refusing to conceive due to a build up of physical deficiencies. The body simply cannot produce offspring after repeated generational declines. This was proven in a ten-year study by Dr. Pottenger which concluded in 1942 where he experimented with the effects of diet on groups of cats. He showed that after generational degeneration, the cats were unable to reproduce.

To learn more about the cause and cures for various ailments, Dr. Joel Fuhrman's book, *Eat to Live*, is probably the best overall resource I can recommend. Organizationally, Hallelujah Acres has a swath of amazing resources of which, *Eat To Live*, is numbered. *The China Study* by Dr. T. Colin Campbell is another wonderful resource and is especially useful for analytical types (like me) who really want delve into the science. *The China Study* is thorough and scientific, but written to be easily understood by anyone. Campbell discusses the diseases that are directly associated with the western, which are heavy in animal protein, by contrasting it to the plant-based Chinese diet. If you want to cure yourself from ever being tempted to taste another bite of anything that came from an animal, then The China Study would certainly be worth a few hours of your time.

It is nice to know that in the midst of all this you can begin to experience wonderful results almost immediately with even some simple changes to your habits.

Pick Your Ailment, Pick Your Recipe.

If you desire one of the following types of ailments, then simply follow the respective recipe and you will be well on your way.

OPTION A: Long-term debilitating disease.

If you have a deep desire to have an attractive nurse doting over your failing body while you lay in a hospital bed, suffering from complications because of a long-term debilitating disease, then you simply need to consume as much animal protein as possible. All animal protein is harmful to the body, including organically grown and grass-fed, as well as the really nasty stuff filled with chemicals and growth hormones. Even dairy contains more than enough pus-filled animal protein to greatly assist in the damage of your God-made physical body. I will discuss the reasons why I don't believe we were intended to consume animals. As well, the recommended resources section at the end of the book has numerous resources you can reference for this topic.

OPTION B: Short-term sickness, cold, flu or other illness.

If sickness is the frequent and standing excuse to miss work, school, church, or anything else on your schedule you would simply need to consume as much refined simple sugar in as many forms as possible. This can come in the form of sugary drinks, highly refined and processed foods, or many other sources of simple sugars. Consuming loads of sugar also comes with other attributes such as massive mood swings, headaches, energy surges and bonks, and of course, obesity.

OPTION C: Obesity.

I have a dear friend who once confessed that she gained weight years prior because she didn't want to be constantly confronted by men with their plans and schemes. If you, too, would like to avoid being attractive to others or yourself, and you think that gluttony of food would be an easy remedy, then don't fear: the solution is at hand. You can simply allow the majority of your diet to be processed and packaged foods. In so doing, you will bypass your body's natural ability to satiate the strongest of appetites once nutritional satisfaction is achieved. This will certainly do the trick, and before long you will be readily gaining pounds.

CHAPTER ELEVEN

What Do I Eat?

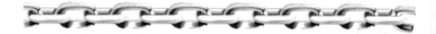

The best food we can consume is raw, fresh, organic produce in as much variety as possible. I believe that we were made to eat produce. I have not come to this conclusion blindly, however. Each of us has unique lives, regions, cultural biases, etc. We have circumstances, and situations that simply can't be lumped into some general teaching for all. It is important to understand that there *is* one perfect diet (conceptually) for all of us, but that there are nuances according to our individual situations and circumstances that we need to consider as we make changes.

To begin, one thing we need to look at is our willingness to accept and adopt change. If we aren't willing, then this could serve as a stumbling block to our success and may slow our progress. This goes back to the discussion about the vices we choose and our ability to see them and choose something other than the things that keep us in chains.

It is critical to realize that I am writing this with many years of implementation experience in my own life. Sometimes I struggled and sometimes I succeeded.

I like to explain it like this: changing your diet to a fully healthy diet is not an overnight decision. It takes time and can be difficult because you are actually changing your mind, which takes time.

If you think of the difference between a dimmer switch and a regular on/off light switch, it will serve as a guidepost for this example.

If you try to jump all the way to a perfect diet immediately then that would be like the regular light switch. It is possible, I suppose, but could be difficult because of the support structure you need to build and the education that you need to develop to succeed in this new environment.

It is common to start with simply cutting out some of the really harmful items such as animal protein and excitotoxins. At the same time you may add some raw, fresh, organic food such as salads and juicing. From there you can play with the mix of raw vs. cooked food as it could take several years to get to the goal of eating primarily raw.

Along the way you will experience things based on what your personal laboratory is telling you it likes. It could be flavors or smells or the way you feel after you eat or drink something. Your body will talk to you very clearly. Listen.

a) Maintain an open mind to change, realizing that what you have been taught previously may not have been truth.

b) Make small, incremental changes with stoic focus on long-term benefits and the eventual culmination of all your steps into a great big, wonderful result.

c) Never stop feeding your mind with good teachings from those you have a reason to trust.

Once you understand the key elements of a healthy diet, you will find that it is very simple to continue to make incremental improvements.

See the resource section of this book for more information on recipes and additional media resources that will help you stay on the critical education path necessary to motivate you.

Below are some great examples of raw foods that we can enjoy:

Beverages . Freshly extracted fruit and vegetable juices are great. Try to drink distilled water with added minerals, if possible.

Dairy Alternatives . Fresh almond milk, creamy banana milk, as well as frozen banana, strawberry or blueberry "fruit creams."

Fruit . All fresh fruit; as well as unsulphured organic dried fruit. Limit consumption to no more than fifteen percent of daily food intake.

Grains. Soaked oats, millet, raw muesli, dehydrated granola, dehydrated crackers, and raw ground flax seed.

Beans. Raw green beans, raw peas, sprouted garbanzo beans, sprouted lentils, and sprouted mung beans.

Nuts and Seeds . Raw almonds, sunflower seeds, macadamia nuts, walnuts, raw almond butter, or tahini.

Oils and Fats . Extra virgin olive oil, coconut oil, coconut butter, grapeseed oil, raw unrefined flax oil and avocados.

Seafoods. Raw, as often found in sushi.

Seasonings. Fresh or dehydrated herbs, garlic, sweet onions, parsley, cayenne pepper, sea salt, and toxin-free seasonings.

Soups . Raw soups

Sweets . Fresh or frozen, all fruit smoothies, raw fruit pies with nut/date crusts, date-nut squares, etc.

Vegetables . All raw vegetables.

Below are examples of cooked foods we may enjoy:

Beverages . Caffeine-free herbal teas and cereal-based coffee-like beverages, along with bottled organic juices.

Dairy . Non-dairy cheese, rice milk, and organic butter (use all sparingly).

Fruit . Stewed and unsweetened frozen fruits.

Grains . Whole-grain cereals, breads, muffins, pasta, brown rice, millet, etc.

Beans. Lima, aduki, black, kidney, navy, pinto, red, and white beans.

Oils . Mayonnaise made from cold-pressed oils. Non-dairy.

Seafoods. Halibut, tuna, salmon, prawns, etc.

Seasonings . Sea Salt.

Soups . Soups made from scratch without fat, dairy, or table salt.

Sweeteners . Raw, unfiltered honey, rice syrup, unsulphured molasses, stevia, carob, pure maple syrup, date sugar.

Vegetables. Steamed or wok-cooked fresh or frozen vegetables, baked white or sweet potatoes, squash, etc.

While this list may appear a bit limiting at first, there are hundreds, if not thousands, of exciting recipes that meet these criteria. I regularly have people comment there is simply no way they could eat as I do. The reality is that they are the ones who are living the limited lives. They only eat what they were raised eating or what the local eateries serve. These people generally visit just a handful of restaurants, and order the very same thing nearly every time. Combine that with the fact that they have only a few recipes at home that they make with any regularity, and then tell me who has the variety and who doesn't.

To give you an example, on Tuesday evenings, for eight years, we host an open, healthy food-preparation evening in our home for our community, and we made 150-200 new recipes each year. Think about this for a minute. There are literally tens of thousands of different types of fruits and vegetables, so many that you could eat several a day each day for your entire life and never repeat any of them. Combining these produce varieties with herbs and spices will yield even more options. Even if you spent your entire life trying to experience every combination you would not even begin to tap into the variety that is available.

I often say I have eaten many more foods I don't like since the change in diet than I did before, not because of lack of variety but because of the massive increase in variety!

Below is a graphic showing the limited the typical western diet flavor spectrum.

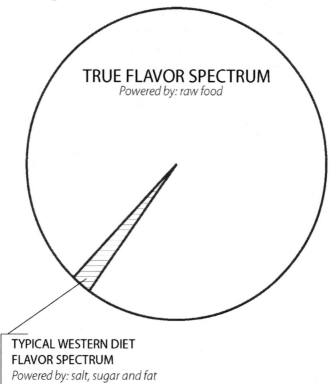

TRUE FLAVOR SPECTRUM
Powered by: raw food

TYPICAL WESTERN DIET
FLAVOR SPECTRUM
Powered by: salt, sugar and fat

I've indicated the limited percentage that our culture accepts on the flavor spectrum to the limitless variety as intended by our creative and wonderful Creator God.

There are some wild flavors out there! One of my favorite fruits is found in Thailand called a durian. It has the foulest smell imaginable but it tastes and feels like custard when eaten. Our family is divided in opinion about that fruit. Nikki and Gabe won't touch it while Jake, Farrell, and I sit in the back yard (because it stinks so badly) and plow through it. Guess what? That is just one type of food and it wasn't mixed with anything. We have the opportunity to make billions of different recipes and even more variations of those recipes. Food variety in this world is endless so don't let one dislike end your curiosity. If you try something and don't like it then just say so and move on to one of the seven billion other options available.

Whoa. I feel better now that I've got that out of the way. I hope you are encouraged when you see the variety designed for our diets. Remember that our food is our fuel. If you feel like you need more variety then seek out great recipes and find ways to get creative with sauces and spices. You can also make a salad with the very same ingredients but with each of the ingredients cut differently and the salad will take on a whole new feel and flavor.

CHAPTER TWELVE

A Typical Healthy Day

When transitioning to a new nutritional lifestyle it can be hard to imagine what a daily food routine will look like. There is opportunity to try different raw foods or cooked dishes, but here is an example of a typical healthy day.

Breakfast
Upon rising, you won't be famished so take it slow. I enjoy a fresh juice in the morning and always include something green. The morning juice is often a fruity one and sometimes I will juice some greens and mix it with a fruit/ice smoothie in the blender. It is best to avoid cooked food or foods containing fiber in the morning as the digestive system is waking up and needs to move smoothly.

Mid-Morning
Drink some fresh juice or eat a small bowl of juicy, fresh fruit. In our home, the breakfast and mid-morning snack often swap places depending upon what we desire.

Lunch

Lunch should always be a raw vegetable salad or raw fruit lunch. It is best to emphasize vegetables over fruit, as the natural sugar content is higher in fruit. Our family really enjoys fish tacos or veggie fajitas if we dine out. Lunch is preferably an all-raw meal but again, it may take some time to get to that point. Do not force the changes—continue the education and move as you feel your mind and your body are ready. Lean on the recommended list of foods as your knowledge increases through your experience.

Mid-Afternoon

Fresh juice and smoothies are always great options. A sliced cucumber is a favorite of mine. Dip it in fresh lemon juice, hummus, or tahini. A piece of fruit is also a quick and easy option.

Supper/Dinner

The evening is a hotly debated topic for those traveling this healthier path. Well, the debate is really with the habits of our culture and the realities of what is best for us. One change that we have made is that we don't generally eat dinner. We did for years but we got to a point where we realized that we had high-quality sleep followed by feeling refreshed in the morning. I know that omitting dinner is not popular but it is what we feel works best for us after years of education and experience.

Early in our transition we would eat large green salads comprised of leaf lettuce along with a variety of vegetables. Do not use head lettuce as it has very little nutritional value. We would also enjoy some cooked food such as baked potato, brown rice, legumes, steamed veggies, whole grain pasta, a veggie sandwich on whole grain bread, baked sweet potato, squash, or any other type of whole grain or vegetable.

Occasionally we would switch raw foods to dinnertime and eat cooked food at lunch.

If possible, avoid eating late. If you want to eat something, be sure to keep it raw such as a piece of fresh fruit or a glass of freshly extracted juice.

As I talk through this, realize that I am many years into this experience. If you are at day one, all of this may seem incredibly foreign to you. Remember that this is a transition. You transitioned from breast milk as a baby into the diet regiment as recommended and practiced by your family. You can transition again, but give yourself some time. Don't get into a spike-and-slide routine where you make big changes and then slide back to where you were. That is a recipe for failure. Make incremental and sustainable changes you can live with, adjust to, and feel like are an advantage and not like a punishment. Always keep an eye on your next incremental change or improvement.

It took us a long time to really get into a regular rhythm with juicing. I believe that our transition would have happened much faster had we adopted a good daily discipline of this sooner.

For the kids, we began them on a dehydrated green juice powder when they were only a few months old. As babies, we would dip their pacifiers in the green powder and they loved it. Now they all really enjoy our juices and they actually make many of them.

In the mornings the kids enjoy chopped cantaloupe or honeydew melon—their favorites! I like to whip up a bowl of raw breakfast cereal; recipe is as follows:

- 1 chopped peach
- ½ chopped apple
- 10 raspberries
- ¼ cup raisins
- Small handful of frozen blueberries
- ¼ cup shredded coconut, large shreds
- ¼ cup chopped walnuts

- ¼ cup puffed corn (we use puffed millet also—both sparingly, of course)
- ½-¾ cup fresh almond milk

Lunch is generally a light raw salad most days. For a long time I used to gorge on a huge salad at lunch because it was what I needed to feel full. I crave great salads every day and it is so wonderful to crave what is good for you!

We found along the way that we slept better at night if we avoided cooked foods in the evening. Ideally, we would finish our eating for the day in the early afternoon but that is still a challenge for us, mainly due to our schedules. See, even I still have my eyes on the next step. I just feel so much better on an empty stomach or a bit of a hungry feeling than always feeling topped off, full or bloated.

It is interesting to point out here that Dr. Joel Fuhrman notes in *Eat to Live* that few of us ever actually experience true hunger. I can confirm now that this is actually true. I enjoy the feeling of being slightly hungry but also enjoy eating just enough to satisfy that hunger rather than gorging or gluttony. Most of us eat out of habit, and we build an unreasonable appetite due to our poor eating habits and choices. Fuhrman comments on this appetite anomaly in people who consume a primarily plant-based diet:

> *Even when they delay eating and get very hungry, they no longer experience stomach cramps, headaches, or fatigue accompanying their falling blood sugar. They merely get hungry and they enjoy this new sensation of hunger in the mouth and throat, which makes food taste better than ever. Many of my patients have told me that they enjoy this new sensation; they like being able to be in touch with true hunger and the pleasure of satisfying it.*

The one point I want to emphasis is that it does not require any precise measuring of calories or specific diet to maintain a thin, muscular weight. It only requires that you eat healthy food and be guided by true hunger.

Now remember, it took me several years to get to this point. It is not something you should feel great pressure about achieving quickly.

As time has passed I have been surprised to find that the less cooked food I eat, the better I feel. I still crave it sometimes and I do eat a bit of cooked food, but I always feel better on fresh, raw, organic, living, and whole food. The cooked food is included in our diet more as a transitional food than anything else. An all-raw diet is best for optimal health but certainly not necessary. The reality is that we consume more nutrients than we actually need when we eat primarily raw, whole foods therefore consuming some cooked food is not detrimental to our overall goal of maintaining optimal health.

Interestingly, even a couple of years ago I would have balked if someone was to tell me that someday I would be eating nearly all raw, whole foods. Education over time has changed my opinion of a raw food diet. My desire now is to eat fuel that is going to make me feel the best, and if it is raw food then that is what I want the most. If I ever progress to an all-raw diet then I welcome that change.

I am, however, not interested in sacrificing relationships or even moments of joy with people over food. If someone were to invite our family over for dinner, worked hard on the meal, and unknowingly included something that we don't normally eat, I would most likely respectfully eat some of it. The exceptions to this statement would be that if it contained animal products. Then I would avoid as much of it as possible, if not all together, and if it contained excitotoxins of any kind then I would not eat it. These items are the chief offenders in my opinion, and they do cause immediate problems for many people, certainly for someone who is very clean internally as I am.

Fortunately, we nearly always have opportunities to discuss alternative food plans with those with whom we socialize. It is often a welcome learning experience for them to try something new with us or as they prepare for us. The point here is that food is designed to bring us together in relationship as much as it is to feed and nourish our bodies. Using food to avoid being in community or using food incorrectly within relationships would be wrong. Food is an integral component of life, not the point.

Without careful planning, however, socializing can undermine eating habits. My family tends to be a lot more flexible away from home than we are at home. This is because we decided we were going to make things more simple at home in terms of choices by not stocking things in the house that are not raw. We want to be as vigilant as possible at home in our eating, snacking, and food choices. This is the core because it is the primary place we eat. Furthermore, it enables us to feel as though we are testing our willpower when we travel or eat out. Clearly, eating away from home is going to be more of a challenge, and actually impossible to accurately know for sure what you are consuming.

I rarely order a salad when eating out. If I do, it can be considered a huge complement because I am usually so dissatisfied with restaurant salads that I just avoid them all together. There are few places where I can get a good one. The biggest single criteria we look for when considering eating in a new place is whether they use any sort of excitotoxin (such as MSG). If so, we won't eat there. The second consideration is if they are flexible in taking their standard menu items and modifying them a bit. If we can get past these two then we are likely headed to sit down and share some time together as a family. As a side note, we would do research online if we were planning a meeting at a restaurant. Researching the establishment's accommodations can avoid an uncomfortable situation.

My advice for eating out is to take a scan over the menu to try to ascertain what they have in the kitchen. Assuming they are really flexible, you can mix and match and put together a really fun, unique meal. My favorite times are when I can just ask the waiter to request the chef "feed us" a nice vegan meal. I usually top this with a request that they avoid pasta because that seems to be a quick solution for some amateur purveyors of the kitchen. If they are comfortable with a whole food diet or a vegan diet then they can often have a lot of fun with this. I think it would be great fun to create individual dishes for customers based on their food preferences. Maybe someday someone will come up with a restaurant like this. Wouldn't that be fun to do as a chef?

One of the things that needs to be avoided is using our busy life schedule to avoid eating healthfully; in other words, to eat out more as an excuse to binge rather than planning the time to go home and enjoy something more full of life. We often feel guilty for eating out, as well, because we have so much live food at home that has a definite shelf life. It is really tough for us to keep up with eating it all, so some does go to waste.

The biggest point I hope you have gained from this discussion of a healthy day is that a day of good eating, in our culture, does require preparation. Once you get into a healthy eating rhythm, however, you are less likely to feel like forethought is such a chore. You will also find that when you stock your home with good, healthy, fresh, whole foods, you have more of a tendency to grab things that are good for you when snacking.

I hope you have hundreds of happy, healthy days ahead!

CHAPTER THIRTEEN

WARNING! Steer Clear...

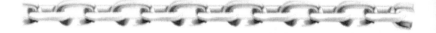

My hope is that this book is not characterized as a book with a bunch of restrictions. In fact, I nearly omitted this section altogether because I feel it is much more important that you focus on what you can do rather than what you should not do. In other words, you can be very successful in just doing the right things right, for the right reasons, rather than focusing on avoiding the wrong things and giving yourself a bad attitude and miserable disposition.

With that said, I am going to be very brief here and give you a list of the items you should avoid and the reasons why. I also want you to see how these apply to my recipes for disease, illness, and obesity.

> The foods listed below create most of the physical problems we experience and are not a part of a typical day for me. To have real health, eliminate them from your diet as quickly as possible with an emphasis on the two categories following this list.

Foods to Be Avoided

Beverages. Alcohol (enjoy sparingly), coffee, carbonated beverages and soft drinks, all artificial fruit drinks (including sports drinks), and all commercial juices containing preservatives, salt, and sweeteners.

Dairy. All milk, cheese, eggs, ice cream, whipped toppings, and non-dairy creamers.

Fruit. Canned and sweetened fruits, non-organic dried fruits.

Grains. Refined, bleached flour products, cold breakfast cereals, and white rice.

Meats. Beef, pork, fish, chicken, turkey, hamburgers, hot dogs, bacon, sausage, etc.

Nuts & Seeds. All roasted and/or salted seeds and nuts.

Oils. All lard, margarine, shortenings, and anything containing hydrogenated oils.

Seasonings. Table salt and most prepackaged seasonings.

Soups. All canned, packaged, or creamed soups containing dairy products.

Sweets. All refined white or brown sugars, sugar syrups, chocolate, candy, gum, cookies, donuts, cakes, pies, or other products containing refined sugars or artificial sweeteners.

Vegetables. All canned vegetables containing added sodium or preservatives, or vegetables fried in oil.

Once you have stopped eating the foods that will harm your health and started eating the foods that will enhance your health, you may experience some unpleasant symptoms of detoxification. If you do, remain steadfast! This means you are getting rid of toxins that have been stored in your body.

This list is extensive. Therefore, if I were to distinguish two foods as the most critical to eliminate, I would select animal products and excitotoxins.

Animal products of any kind would be one that I would simply avoid all together. Dr. T. Colin Campbell explains, in detail, why animal products are so bad for the human body in his book, *The China Study*. It has to do with the protein and how it is processed in our bodies. It is really bad for our bodies as it leads to many of the western diseases we commonly experience as a culture. Dr. Joel Fuhrman in *Eat to Live* confirms this, and many life stories along with hundreds of scientific studies also corroborate this fact. This includes dairy, quite significantly because dairy includes the animal protein that is the chief contributor to physical ailments. The studies around fish and seafood are rather vague, however. It seems the protein in these is not as severely problematic as is the toxic load from the heavy metals often found in them. I ate some fish during the first couple of years of the lifestyle change but it was infrequent and in small portions. *Eat to Live* has a helpful chart showing which fish are more likely to contain more heavy metals and therefore should be avoided.

Excitotoxins of all kinds are also extremely dangerous. Much of the preeminent work on excitotoxins is by Dr. Russell Blaylock, documented in his book, *Excitotoxins*. Much of what I have to share is from his work as well as from first-hand experience with excitotoxin chemical poisoning. Because I know you want to know what an excitotoxin is, I will provide a brief overview here but if you want to know details then refer to Blaylock's book.

What is an excitotoxin? An excitotoxin is an amino acid. Our bodies use a lot of amino acids regularly. The problem is that there are ways of creating amino acids in such a manner that they zoom past the protective blood-brain barrier and wreak havoc on our brain neurons (receptors). These "bad" amino acids are named excitotoxins because of their effect on human neurology. The excitotoxin amino acid travels to the receptors in the brain that control the "feel good" signals, which act like gates. The excitotoxin holds open the gate to the receptor while calcium rushes in to cause the receptor to fire in rapid succession, sending a "feel good" signal elsewhere in the brain. Zinc and magnesium are designed to hold the gate closed in certain circumstances, but a deficiency in these minerals is common and thus leaves the receptors even more vulnerable. In other words, we are tricked into thinking that whatever we just did (or ate) was good for us and pleasurable. Soon after, the receptors (neurons) effected by the excitotoxin die. Here is what Dr. Blaylock says about the effects of the excitotoxins:

> *"When neurons are exposed to these substances, they become very excited and fire their impulses very rapidly until they reach a state of extreme exhaustion. Several hours later these neurons suddenly die, as if the cells were excited to death. As a result, neuroscientists have dubbed this class of chemicals 'excitotoxins.'"*

Clearly excitotoxins are something we should avoid, but where are they found? Some of the common names would be MSG or hydrolyzed protein. The problem is that many people know about the negative effects of MSG, so food manufacturers have resorted to creating new, similar substances and conveniently renaming them something else. Below is a reference list compiled by Dr. Joel Fuhrman, from his book, *Eat To Live*:

The following always contain an excitotoxin:

Autolyzed Plant Protein
Autolyzed yeast
Calcium caseinate
Gelatin
Glutamate
Glutamic acid
Hydrolyzed Plant Protein (HPP)
Hydrolyzed Vegetable Protein (HVP)
Monopotassium glutamate
Monosodium glutamate
MSG
Senomyx (wheat extract labeled as artificial flavor)

Sodium caseinate
Textured protein
Vegetable protein extract
Yeast extract
Yeast food or nutrient

The following commonly contain an excitotoxin:
Algae, phytoplankton, sea vegetable, wheat or barley grass powders
Amino acids (as in Bragg's liquid amino acids and chelated to vitamins)
Annatto
Barley malt
Bouillon
Broth
Caramel flavoring (coloring)
Carrageenan
Citric acid (when processed from corn)
Corn syrup and corn syrup solids, high fructose corn syrup
Cornstarch fructose (made from corn)
Dough conditioners
Dry milk solids
Enzyme modified proteins
Fermented proteins
Flowing agents
Gluten and gluten flour
Gums (guar and vegetable)
Lecithin
Lipolyzed butterfat
"Low" or "No Fat" items
Malt Extract or Flavoring
Malted barley (flavor)
Maltodextrin, dextrose, dextrates
Milk powder
Modified food starch
Natural chicken, beef, or pork flavoring "seasonings"
Natural flavors, flavors, flavoring
Pectin

Protease
Protease enzymes
Protein fortified milk
Protein powders: whey, soy, oat, rice (as in protein bars shakes and body building drinks)
Reaction flavors
Rice syrup or brown rice syrup
Soy sauce or extract
Soy protein
Soy protein isolate or concentrate
Spice
Stock
Ultra-pasteurized dairy products
Wheat, rice, corn, or oat protein
Whey protein isolate or concentrate
Whey protein or whey
Yeast nutrients
Anything enriched or vitamin enriched
Anything protein fortified

If that list isn't scary enough, Dr. Blaylock indicates that some excitotoxins such as aspartate and L-cysteine can be added to foods without labeling under FDA rules. If you are a smoker, you should also know that some cigarettes now contain excitotoxins, and it is conceivable they could pass through the absorptive surfaces of lung tissue and enter the blood stream. That's a little more motivation to eat a plant!

This is basically the self-administered regime that I have applied to my life with great success. Of course, through the years, I have grown in my understanding and have expanded the list of things I avoid mainly out of choice rather than feeling like it was something I had to do. When I made progress in my health, I didn't feel as good when I ate certain things. Pasta is a good example. I can't remember when I last had more than a bite of pasta, but I know after I did I felt like I had a terrible weight in my stomach. It was bad and I simply decided pasta was no longer for me in any significant quantity. Another example I like to share is my story about dropping the super-sized French fry habit. After I began the diet change, I chose to continue an infrequent McDonald's French fry habit. This continued about once or twice per quarter for a couple of years. The last time was the day I sat in the parking lot, chowing down on the fresh hot fries, and then I realized that I didn't really enjoy the flavor all that much. In fact, my mouth was a bit sticky afterwards and I can't say I felt great after eating them. For me, that was all it took. I wasn't strict about it along the way nor did I beat myself up for doing this. After all, they are vegan! The point here is that in due time you will achieve the goals you set out for, but it will take some time, with focus and diligence.

It is also important to remember to think about what you can do rather than going too far down this path of all that you are bound from. There are more options than any of us will ever be able to explore and experience. Find the freedom in your lifestyle instead of focusing on the restrictions.

CHAPTER FOURTEEN

Supplements & Complements

It may be helpful for a period of time (and possibly for a longer duration depending upon your situation) to combine a healthy diet with some supplements. Through a healthy diet you will get vital nutrients, which will help boost your immune system, as well as provide other health support.

Greens:

It is critical for us to get a large amount of greens in our diet. If you are unable or if you just want a boost, then using a high quality, clean label green powdered juice is a good option and something we did for many years.

Carrot/Vegetable Juice

Freshly extracted carrot/vegetable juice made from large organic juicing carrots and leafy green vegetables is extremely important in meeting daily nutritional needs. Carrots are the richest source of beta-carotene, the precursor of vitamin A (which the body can easily absorb), plus it provides a wealth of other nutritional benefits.

If you do not have a juicer to make your own fresh carrot/vegetable juice, you can use convenient juice powders as substitutes.

Fiber Cleanse

A good herbal fiber cleanse can help cleanse the colon, restore normal bowel activity, ensure timely and efficient elimination of toxins from the body, and more—a must for achieving optimal health.

A diet rich in fibrous produce can also produce great results in cleaning out your digestive track but it is helpful to take an effective supplement to assist the process.

Vitamin B12

Those following a plant-based diet should consider taking a supplement to ensure an adequate level of Vitamin B12 in the body, as this nutrient is not readily found in a primarily-vegan diet. Adequate levels of B12 help the body to do the following: prevent anemia, regulate red blood cell formation, form healthy cells, metabolize fats and carbohydrates, utilize iron, and prevent nerve damage.

The vitamins B6 and Folic Acid provide related health benefits, such as metabolizing protein, forming hemoglobin, and decreasing neural tube defects. We combined B12 with B6 and Folic Acid into a vegetarian sublingual tablet to help you get the best 1-2-3 nutritional health punch this combination can deliver. For those who are pregnant, this combination is a must for your health and that of your child.

Fish Oil

A good fish oil supplement will contribute to the necessary nutrients needed for optimal health. A high quality blend of oils, will give you the essential omega-3 and omega-6 fatty acids that the body needs to achieve and maintain good health. Current research also indicates that men dealing with prostate cancer may be well served by using freshly ground flax seed to meet their essential fat needs.

Sunshine

Each sunny day, get some sunshine (at lest fifteen minutes) on as much of the skin as possible. The sun is exceptionally important in the production of vitamin D, which is critical for strong bones and muscles, a healthy immune system, and more.

Exercise

Exercising every day for a minimum of thirty minutes is extremely important—it helps you stay physically fit and releases toxins from the body. Doing a combination of aerobic, resistance, and stretching exercises will help maximize your body's cardiovascular condition, strength, and flexibility. When first beginning an exercise regimen, doing a stretching and fast walking program is a good place to start.

To learn more about the path I took to get healthy and fit with exercise, get a copy of my *5-Minute Workout* book.

I consider greens to be mandatory for people consuming the typical western diet, or even those eating exceptionally healthfully. There are several reasons, but generally because it is the most nutrient-dense and most wonderful food on the planet. We cannot get perfect food even if we are eating all organic whole foods.

If you refer to Dr. Joel Fuhrman's book, *Eat to Live*, you will see a nutrient density chart. The chart shows low-density foods such as refined sweets, refined oils, refined grains, cheese, and dairy at less then five points of a possible 100. Notice that nothing on the nutrient density chart scoring above fifty is any color other than green. I think this is a great indication from a scientific position that the more we emphasize green foods in our diet, the healthier our bodies will be.

CHAPTER FIFTEEN

Living In Community

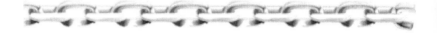

Educating yourself and eating well are excellent components of a healthy lifestyle. Equally important, however, but often overlooked is the benefit of living in community.

There are generally two areas of concern I see when observing American society. First, I see that people are growing apart in a culture that is becoming increasingly separate. Though technological improvements may seem to bring connection, they actually more often undermine real relationships and community.

Secondly, I see that we tend to use community as a crutch for living in unhealthy ways. This is not limited to diet, but we certainly tend to be gluttonous when we meet. The heart behind serving each other sumptuous food is wonderful, but wouldn't it be thoughtful if we took the time to think more holistically about more than just how the food will taste for our guests, but also about the impact to the body? We tend to set negative examples rather than positive ones for each other. We need to challenge each other to live for the right reasons. Again, food is just one piece of a bigger equation here.

When we do meet together, we share our gifts, our experiences, and our talents. When we stay alone or segregate ourselves, we tend to keep the lights low and huddle around making excuses for why we are not doing the things we enjoy – the things we dream of doing but just never do for some reason. My challenge here is for you to get in a community of people you can grow with. If you don't see a community you can join, then lead!

Years ago, we realized we needed a community, so we began hosting weekly classes in our church. After a year, we got fed up with the low attendance and stopped. It was just too much work and we didn't see any practical point of continuing. We were not building community and therefore the community was not growing. After a few weeks, my mom came to us and asked if we would start it up again but in our home. It was a great idea—much easier. And guess what? People showed up! Now we have a packed house nearly every Tuesday evening for a nutritionally educational dinner. We ask for a five-dollar donation for those who can afford it, and we usually try 150-200 new recipes a year—some we like and others we don't. When we are traveling, others will host in our home in our absence. It is a wonderful community and we have met hundreds of people over the years.

The point is that you simply will not be successful with this if you are attempting to be like an island instead of in a community. We are designed to fellowship (to share life together). Remember that life happens when we are together!

One final point I want to make about community and the Tuesday night food prep is that, although we get fifteen to forty-five people on any given Tuesday evening, we would still do it if it was just my family. Seriously, it is really enjoyable for just a few of us to come together and share life. The kids love the kitchen, and it is a wonderful time to experience food and enjoy some time together catching up. It is also a very comfortable setting for people to visit and peek into our real lives. Our food serves as a wonderful gateway to build relationships with people, eventually allowing us to help, support, and love them to a better life. It is not uncommon that we find ourselves helping people physically, and that in turn leads to the more important work of helping them grow personally. This only happens when we meet together and build relationships. This is community and we love it!

Living Counter-Culturally

Whenever you do something counter-cultural, you are more than likely right!

You may be surprised to hear that Nikki and I received only two home dinner invitations during the ten-year period after I was diagnosed. Was this because we had recently gotten married, started having kids, diagnosed with cancer, or because we ate some funky diet that no one really understood? The answer seemed obvious. It was partly because all the changes in our lives seriously impacted the friendships we had. However, most of it was due to the fact we just didn't eat along the lines of our culture. We believe people chose to avoid it for two reasons. First, it was because they didn't want a spotlight illuminating their diet choices; and second, because they just didn't know what food to make or how to prepare it.

This could have been discouraging for us but we were so busy having people over to our place that we really didn't even notice it until several years had passed. We then made a conscious choice to begin attempting to reach out even more to build some more of these vital relationships. We found that once people got to know us and understood why we live the way we do, they became very interested in learning more about it. Sound familiar? This lines up perfectly with how we are to show people the love of God, right?

Living counter-culturally is fun. Being normal is boring! During most of my childhood people called me weird (what was up with that?). I would go home upset, and my mom confirmed it by telling me that "I was not weird—I was just different." Being different somehow made me feel better at the time. As I look back, though, my mom was right on the mark. She taught me a great lesson by confirming I was actually different and that was okay. We are all different. We are all uniquely made. We all have a special combination of attributes that make us, well…us. Isn't it nice to know, however, that we have a loving God who supports, encourages, and loves each of us in the very same way? And, that same Creator made a path for each of us that is perfect for physical health and healing. Find it. Live it. Enjoy it!

CHAPTER SIXTEEN

Lighten Up!

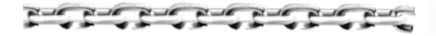

Contrary to what you may think, this chapter isn't primarily about weight loss and you won't find a chapter in the book that specifically addresses weight loss. I deemphasize the topic intentionally. As a culture we are too focused on the wrong things, often blinding us to what is important. We fail to see valuable information or pursue education entirely. Had I titled this chapter "Education," you might have skipped it because that is the way our culture is programmed.

About fifty years ago, when C.S. Lewis wrote *The Screwtape Letters*, he accurately predicted one of the problems with a democratic society. Despite all of the successes of our democratic republic, the freedom found in our society has enabled mankind's propensity to avoid what we need—education.

In section two Lewis writes:

For "democracy" or the "democratic spirit" (diabolical sense) leads to a nation without great men, a nation mainly of sub-literates, full of the cocksureness which flattery breeds on ignorance, and quick to snarl or whimper at the first hint of criticism. And that is what Hell wishes every democratic people to be. For when such a nation meets in conflict a nation where children have been made to work at school, where talent is placed in high posts, and where ignorant mass are allowed no say at all in public affairs, only one result is possible.

C.S. Lewis had the same concern I have, and one I believe we are currently witnessing in western culture. We are more concerned about our comfort than we are about our fundamental future. We think more about what's going on today than we do about preparing a better place for tomorrow.

Our shortsightedness plays out in our lack of desire for education. As a culture, we are trained to "do school" when we are little. Education beyond K-12 is generally optional. We largely attend college to get a degree in some career field, but beyond that, there's really no concern for continuous on-going education.

The chief issue is that it seems we value our comfort and our vices over our responsibility to stray from the current for the sake of the future. If we had a healthy respect for the responsibility that is on our shoulders then we would have less apathy and entitlement and more action, indignation, and entrepreneurship.

The forefathers of this great country never ceased pursuing education and discussing great thought. I would suggest that the state of most modern citizens would have quite literally made them ill. As a veteran, I often wonder if the ultimate price that so many soldiers paid was at least partly in vain. Our second president, John Adams, strongly believed in the value of education.

Laws for the liberal education of youth, especially for the lower classes of people, are so extremely wise and useful that to a humane and generous mind, no expense for this purpose would be thought extravagant.

I must study politics and war that my sons may have liberty to study mathematics and philosophy. My sons ought to study mathematics and philosophy, geography, natural history, naval architecture, navigation, commerce, and agriculture in order to give their children a right to study painting, poetry, music, architecture, statuary, tapestry, and porcelain.

There are two types of education. One should teach us how to make a living, and the other how to live.

John Adams understood the need for education quite clearly. As a society progresses the ability to enjoy the arts increases. By no means, however, does this eliminate the responsibility of those that go after us from continuing to protect and uphold the necessity of education.

Through research I discovered writings of notable people, including our founding fathers, pertaining to the value of education. It's exciting for me to share these quotes with you. These people, so much more distinguished than I, make my points more eloquently than I ever could.

If a nation expects to be ignorant and free, in a state of civilization, it expects what never was and never will be. – Thomas Jefferson, third president of the United States

Education's purpose is to replace an empty mind with an open one. – Malcolm Forbes, publisher of Forbes Magazine

We are shut up in schools and college recitation rooms for ten or fifteen years, and come out at last with a bellyful of words and do not know a thing. – Ralph Waldo Emerson, American essayist

The recipe for perpetual ignorance is: be satisfied with your opinions and content with your knowledge. – Elbert Hubbard, American writer

Life is not divided into semesters. You don't get summers off and very few employers are interested in helping you find yourself. – Bill Gates, co-founder of Microsoft

People will pay more to be entertained than educated. – Johnny Carson, comedian and TV show host

The highest form of ignorance is when you reject something you don't know anything about. – Wayne Dyer, self-help author

I want to motivate you to think about life as a process of learning. These men clearly recognized that education begins with each new day. Day by day, the lessons of life are actually the sessions of our continuing education. You are never too old to take a class online or at the local college. You are welcome to visit local businesses to learn from them, or volunteer to fill a need in your community. You can even learn valuable lessons by sitting with the elderly and listening to their stories about history and personal life choices.

In order for you to be successful in making the right changes that will lead to health and vitality for you, your family, and the future generations of your family, each of us must commit to continuing to allow education to be a vital part of our days. What that looks like for you may be different than for me, but the end result is the same. We will hopefully have a solid grasp on what life is suppose to be lived like on this planet earth in these human bodies and that clarity will assist us in living out the joy and adventure that is intended for each of our lives.

Equally important is the blessing of revelation. Revelations are pure and utter gifts from God. The effect of revelation is no different than true education. The only difference is that we don't have to work for revelation. When you look at the history of our country, and likely many of the people who have surrounded your life, you will no doubt see many people who relied on God for inspiration through revelation. Samuel Adams, George Walton, Benjamin Franklin, and John Hancock, along with all of the founding fathers of this country, kneeled together in prayer on the congressional floors of this great country. Their prayers are documented in the historical records. They understood the value of revelation, and they respected the God who so generously provides it in a way that is difficult for us to fully grasp.

Our lives begin to end when we lose interest in furthering our vision through education and revelation.

Weight Loss & Calories

First of all, we need to gain a proper understanding of this entire topic. We should attempt to be content with our physical body as it is, yet maintain stoic focus on where we are going and where we want to be. What I mean is, do not condemn yourself for your present state. You can't change the choices you made in the past, but you can change what you do today and all the days that still lie ahead. Self-condemnation is unhealthy and can be used to simply create an excuse to slip back into unhealthy patterns.

Secondly, we need to gather a proper understanding of how much we should weigh. I believe this varies between people, but in general it is safe to say we can use a range. I like the tool that Dr. Joel Fuhrman shared in *Eat to Live*:

Women: Approximately ninety-five pounds for the first five feet of height and then four pounds for every inch thereafter. Example: A 5'6" female should weigh approximately 119 pounds.

$$5'4'' \quad 95 + 16 = 111$$

$$5'6'' \quad 95 + 24 = 119$$

Men: Approximately 105 pounds for the first five feet of height and then five pounds for every inch thereafter. Example: A 5'10" male should weight approximately 155 pounds.

$$5'9'' \quad 105 + 45 = 150$$

$$6'0'' \quad 105 + 60 = 165$$

With this information in hand, we can establish some general guidelines for where we should be with our weight; however, worrying about a number on the scale isn't the point. I always maintain that calorie counting is a waste of time. Let's put our focus on the right things and allow the results to land where they may. When you do figure out your weight range using Dr. Fuhrman's numbers, put it in an envelope and never look at it again, because it doesn't matter. Please, if you are one of the many that do need to drop a few pounds, don't get caught in the undercurrent of living for a certain weight. You miss out on the joy today has if you are living for someday. You shouldn't target a certain weight as your goal, but rather a healthy lifestyle. When you do that, your body will naturally respond.

There is no good reason to count calories if you are eating a primarily raw, whole food, or plant-based diet. When you eat a bag of chips, you can consume the entire bag and still be hungry because your stomach did not register any nutrition. It is sifting through what you are eating and it isn't finding anything of real value. Therefore, the signal to stop eating is simply not sent until you begin to feel the uncomfortable pressure of overeating. This is really not good but tends to be the way we eat. We eat what is set before us, right? If we don't feel the pressure then we may opt for something extra or a dessert. Either way, we generally get some sort of feeling of physical fullness. To me, full is simply the absence of a reminder. My whole body will scream at me if I get too hungry. I know what true hunger feels like. Interestingly enough, one would think during times like this that I would need to eat a huge meal to overcome such a loud and annoying call for nourishment. I just need a few bites and it all goes away. It will likely return quickly if I don't eat very much; but because I eat foods that my body recognizes, we are able to communicate with one another freely. It tells me what it needs and I give it something recognizable. It tells me when to stop and I naturally lose interest in eating. Yes, I said, naturally and without thought, I stop eating and walk away from the food. Cool, huh?

Think about a meal as a literal walk through the garden. There would be no plates or forks, right? So, how much would you pick? Well, if you were on a dinner walk, you would hopefully have someone enjoyable with you like your spouse, some friends, or family members. You would walk, talk, and pick whatever you wanted. You would be chiefly focused on food at the beginning because you would be hungry, but then as you lost interest in your food, your focus would turn to each other. You'd continue to walk right past most of the food hanging all around you. There would be no dishes or leftovers. Also, there would be no overeating or counting calories. Wouldn't it be neat to have a garden that you could take dinner walks in, and a family that would want to do it with you? Maybe this is a new restaurant concept...

At some point in the future, after you begin implementing these diet changes, you may want to check that ideal weight envelope—and when you do, it will be fun! I lost about forty pounds in the first year after I made the change in my diet and lifestyle. About four years later, I lost another twenty pounds and now I am fine-tuning my muscle tone and weight. The key to success is enjoying the process, not dreading it.

Cleansing – Frequency

Many people ask, but most don't have the stamina. Everyone wants to know if they poop often enough, and is the consistency correct. If there is some pain or blood, is that normal? (No, it is not normal, if you are wondering.) Interestingly enough, nearly everything you ever need to know about your physical body can be found with close analysis of your stool. So, the thinking on this is most certainly on the right track.

Transfer time is a measurement of the period of time from the beginning point when you eat through to evacuation of the bowels. This includes travel time through the body. The body is like a donut. You could say our digestive system is in our body, but the food that travels through it is never actually inside the body. It is inside the donut hole, sure, but it doesn't actually enter the body. It is just acted upon by the digestive system. It is either hydrated or dehydrated depending upon the stage in the process. So just how long does this process take and how often should it happen?

The digestive system is the tool to provide your body with nourishment. Many people see it as an extraction tool but that isn't the primary function. We wrongly see it as a machine to extract the nutrition from the things that we eat. For example, you eat a hamburger and think that your body will pull the nutrients from the lettuce, tomato, and ketchup, and of course the "ever important" protein from the meat, (that part is a lie in case you don't know yet—refer back to Chapter 8 under "Animal Products"), and then send it into your blood stream and throughout your body for whatever all those various organs need.

Unfortunately, that is the way most of us use the digestive system. Yet, it is actually designed to quickly capture the nutrients, which are chiefly mechanically extracted with our teeth in our mouth where nutrient absorption begins. There is some minor chemical breakdown that happens in our stomach, but not nearly as much as we commonly burden our stomach with. In other words, the right foods provide nutrients that are easily absorbable with our bodies. The stomach, and the rest of the system, doesn't need to take a lot of action to extract the nutrition.

I will use myself as an example since my body has been a living laboratory for ten years. Well, actually forty years if you count all the years I was eating like the billboards tell us to.

I use the bathroom every time I eat. It is a natural reaction for you body to clean out the old and make space for the new. The actual transit time should be well below twenty-four hours. Any guess what the typical transit time is for a westerner's diet? It's about seventy-two hours, or three days. So here is something else to think about: what happens to a bunch of fresh raw produce if you put it in the blender, and then let it sit out at room temperature for twenty-four hours? Not much right? In fact, it will most definitely still contain some life. Now think about the burger. If you blend that up (you will naturally have to add some soda pop so it will blend properly in the blender, right?) and set it out on the counter at room temperature for three days, what is it going to look like or smell like?

The problem is that certain foods make your digestive system sluggish, and it does not push as aggressively as it normally would. This is caused primarily by foods low in fiber. Did you know animal products do not contain a bit of fiber? Fiber is what activates the contractions within your intestines. It keeps things moving through. Produce is full of fiber and water-packed with essential nutrients. The nutrient-packed water is the lifeblood of the plant. The fiber is just the carrier, so wouldn't it make sense that it would cause your intestines to contract and push it through by design?

Your intestines are designed to be a one-way tool. Once the food passes a certain point, toxins and additional water should be added to the intestines, but nothing should be coming from the other direction. If slow-moving food sits in your digestive system for days then it has the opportunity to enable toxins to enter back into the body.

So, how do you increase elimination frequency? Eat more fiber! It will excite your intestines and encourage the movement of much of the muck and pus that builds up from tons of simple carbohydrates and animal protein. It is certainly an easy way to lose a few pounds! Simply consume a raw, plant-based diet for a few days to see the results. There are also some herbs that can help stimulate the bowels into action. Hallelujah Acres has an herbal fiber blend that works really well. If you persist in eating a western diet, then you may consider a periodic cleanse with something like this. I am not promoting consumption of the typical western diet, but this is greatly beneficial if you do.

Since our discussions have landed us in the southern regions of our bodies, some of you may know of or wonder about the cause of rectal itching. It is caused by parasites (more toxins) being forced out during the natural detoxification process. It isn't supposed to last long, but can be expected if you make some improvements in your eating habits as your body begins to cleanse. It is gross, but it should be encouraging to know they are on their way out instead of being allowed to remain.

A diet you will most certainly hear about, if you have not already, is "The Full Plate Diet." I have studied it briefly, but have no affiliation with the organization. What I can say, from what I have seen thus far, is that they are likely going to gain a strong following. Generally they do encourage people to move in a healthy direction. The concern I have is that they don't seem to provide much structure for people who want to go beyond some fairly basic and simple changes. They seem to think people are likely just going to make minor changes, yet continue to live and eat according to our culture. They seem to be making tangible sense of the dimmer vs. light switch I discussed earlier in the book. "The Full Plate Diet" is really based on that methodology, which makes the diet transition very easy. They also do utilize many online social outlets to encourage participants with the support of like-minded people.

CHAPTER SEVENTEEN

Fasting, Feasting & Funny Names

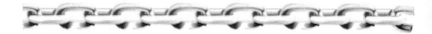

I was recently asked about the Daniel Fast, which is also known as the Daniel Diet.

To begin, here is the verse from the book of Daniel where the diet comes from: "If in ten days, I can look noticeably better, then that is certainly something that deserves a bit more attention."

1) What is the purpose of a "fast?"

Fasting is, biblically speaking, a time for us to get our eyes off of the things of this world and onto God. We could fast from lots of things in our culture, but most tend to think of food when fasting. We could also, without feeling hypocritical, choose to "fast" for physical reasons. The purpose for this fast is generally to rest the body's digestive system and allow cleansing. Some people do this annually for a month or so. I agree that it is a healthy approach, but would not endorse water fasting since the detoxification is often severe and can be dangerous. Fresh juice fasting, or even raw food fasting, is a great way for people who are entrenched in the standard American diet to clean themselves up for a period of time. Ultimately, eating healthfully throughout the year instead of using a fast to clean yourself up or lose a little weight is a better approach.

2) Live the truth... temporarily?

If you go all the way back to creation and ignore what happened after Adam and Eve sinned, you will quickly see what God's "original intent" was for our physical health, healing, and wholeness. He intended us to eat raw produce! Read Genesis 1:29 for His specific assignment in this regard. So here's what God's instruction amounted to: we should eat as much raw, organic produce as we can, all the time. At the same time, given the data we have from the research done by doctors like Dr. Campbell on those who consume animal products, chemically-filled processed foods, and such, it seems to make sense to limit or even eliminate such foods. Doing a cleansing fast for a period of time each year, in my opinion, is worse for your physical body than just eating a more balanced diet all the time, which contains a majority percentage of raw, organic produce. The ups and downs in your system can be difficult and the mental part is deceiving.

By cleansing for a few weeks a year, we give way to the thinking that we can just eat anything we want the rest of the year until the time of the cleansing comes around again and we "sacrifice" for a few weeks. A few bites here, a few pounds there, oh, don't worry, the cleanse will clear it up. Furthermore, we really miss the benefits of living a healthy lifestyle. I was healed of cancer, my wife of irritable bowel syndrome (IBS), and our kids have generally been free of sickness their entire lives. That is not to say there isn't a rare occasion of some bug that comes around, but it is very infrequent, minor in terms of symptoms, never requires a doctor visit, and it is uncommon that we even use any sort of medicine other than a mild pacifier.

In addition, my family's physical bodies are fit and healthy. We feel good about ourselves. Others regularly comment on the beauty of our family. Some stare in astonishment when they see the huge salads our kids regularly consume.

So my encouragement to you would be to look at this as a journey. I would suggest a nice steady growth pattern starting right where you are as a great trajectory. Don't feel like you need to conquer the world this week. But to accomplish this you need to demonstrate something that is uncommon in our culture: self-discipline and commitment. You need to continue to educate your mind and pray for revelation and strength to stay on track. Not making a massive change in the beginning means you need to walk a slight upslope forever. Yes, forever. Think about it. A big change now means that inevitably you will walk a down-slope for the next couple of years back to where you are. Doesn't it make more sense to just start where you are, commit to the journey and begin making changes? You can do it! I know you can.

3) What are all these terms and names for diets?

A *vegetarian* is someone who does not eat animal meat but does consume dairy products.

A *vegan* is a vegetarian who also avoids dairy products.

A *vegish* is a vegan who consumes fish and various types of seafood.

A *pescitarian* is a vegetarian who also consumes fish.

4) What exactly is "feasting?"

Feasting is a common term you may hear. Some use the word to replace the word 'fasting,' but it may mean the same thing. Others use the word because it describes how they feel about food. Fasting seems to have a negative connotation while feasting is more positive and denotes abundance. I have done a forty-day "green coconut feast." There was nothing spiritual about this, per se. I just wanted to experience a lot of greens and see the impact in my life. I didn't eat just green coconuts, by the way. I ate all things green along with as much coconut as I wanted! It truly was a feast, and it was fun to be able to experiment with various unique ingredients.

CHAPTER EIGHTEEN

The Facts

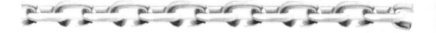

We were created to live healthfully for a long time on limited raw, fresh, organic, vine-ripened produce. We also have the physical ability to sustain ourselves with much less variety than we often think we require. In India, where most of the mangos are grown, you could enjoy a season where you could quite literally eat as many mangos as you want and not begin to make a dent in the resource. The nutrients that come from a particular plant are not altogether unique. Sure, some produce contains increased or decreased amounts of certain nutrients, but it is possible to sustain life on very few of these life-giving nutrients. We see it lived out everyday as people gorge themselves on substances they call food, yet ones that are totally devoid of any nutritional value. Somehow, our bodies are able to maintain themselves even while we provide only little or no high quality, living nutrients.

The majority of the produce on earth dies on the vine. Most of it is never picked, or even looked upon. It will grow and die and the cycle continues. Some blackberry bushes grow near my office. There are thousands of berries on them each year, and I think my kids and I are the only ones who actually eat any of them. We make such a small dent that it is difficult to imagine how many people could actually be enjoying this wonderful fruit. I searched and searched for some facts on how much or what percentage of the world is deficient in food sources, specifically the areas that are deprived of a sufficient supply of food to sustain healthy life. Clearly, the answer for our food shortage problem is to redefine what food is. Could it be that the redefinition of food has already happened and we are relying on a false definition, which is currently causing the shortage in supply? Well, maybe not. It could be that we just have a distribution or logistical problem, but I would venture to guess that we do have a definition problem. If we redefine food back to what it is supposed to be, then we can focus on the simple task of distributing that food. Food is not whatever is possible to compile nor what a manufacture can make a profit on but actually stuff that is designed to bring nutrition or fuel to our living bodies. Living organisms feed off other live things. Food should be defined as fresh, raw, and alive! We can also educate others on how to produce food throughout the world and literally solve the hunger and perceived shortages quickly.

We have expanded our view of the definition of food, and then we have applied inappropriate focus on things that should not be considered food. At the same time, we have ignored the real food that is simply dying on the vine.

A few years ago, I set out to help my kids with a little school project. I thought it would be neat to build a little mobile that showed a couple of planets and how they revolved around each other. I wanted to do something extra special with Earth. My plan was to add a little wire that would spin around Earth, which would be in position to indicate the thickness of the atmosphere. This would be a great demonstration, which would show the actual size of the livable area around Earth.

What I wanted to show was how thick (or thin) the atmosphere is. I thought this would be interesting mainly because I look out at the space and size of the universe, dream about the unknown galaxies, and quite literally live in amazement of the size of creation! When you consider that vast size of the space in which we live, which was specially and specifically designed for us to be sustained, life has more meaning. I wanted to build this little model so it would enable my kids to see how really small that livable space really was. What I found still shocks me to think about to this day.

This amazing globe given to us to thrive upon for our short years is less than 8,000 miles in diameter. The depth of the atmosphere is about 23 miles. As you can imagine, the little six-inch foam ball I intended to use to represent Earth in our mobile made it extremely tough to represent the thickness of the livable space around it. The math calculated that with a six-inch diameter ball (which represented the 8,000 miles in diameter of Earth) the thickness of the atmosphere around our mobile needed to be paper-thin!

This realization took my breath away as I pondered the idea of how small our space really is. Taking this thought a bit further, I found it fascinating that we do not have a visible layer of protection to separate the livable space from space itself. We cannot see the dividing line with our eyes. Why is there just a limited amount of space for us to live? Why is not the entire universe made up of the same properties as the small area we refer to as the atmosphere?

For now, let's take another look at the facts of our existence. There are currently about 6.6 billion people on earth. If were to stack all people closely together we could into a space that is about the size of one quarter of a square mile cube. That means a cube of space that is only one quarter of a mile tall, deep, and wide.

With that understanding, and the size of the earth as previously discussed, does it seem possible for us to have a tremendous, or even measurable, impact on the earth's resources? My point here is not to rail in the face of the "green movement." In fact, I agree with it and drive efficiency on a daily basis, which is really what living green is all about. The idea is that we want to be more efficient, but also to simply create less of a load on the overall system. One of my major talents is, in fact, building processes that ultimately cause more efficient lives and systems. Therefore, I am a big fan of green initiatives. What I don't agree with is marketing companies, governments, and organizations using tools such as this to manipulate us through fear to act in certain ways. Like I said, this is a whole different story, but the point is that we have been fooled, duped, and manipulated in our thinking. On our own, we have walked along ignorantly into the hands of those who stand to gain from our blank stares.

One example of this can be found in the concerns about the ozone layer around the earth. A few decades ago, it became big news that there were potentially dangerous holes in the ozone. The assumption was that we were chemically burning these holes with the excessive factories and use of toxins in our daily lives. The reality is that there were other factors that contributed to these findings. We had just developed the technology to be able to read the density of the ozone, and since there was no meaningful baseline to determine how much the layer had changed, the noted occurrences of thinning in the ozone were treated as a negative. Actually, what was happening was that the ozone layer was performing as it was designed to function by opening, shifting, and closing to allow gases to be released from the atmosphere. Just like our bodies are self-healing, the atmosphere has also been designed to take care of itself. Nevertheless, just like we are seeing with the green movements, self-serving companies will jump on these reports to make the most of them financially.

If you are still in disbelief about the responsibility that companies and government have on our food supply, then read this quote from the CEO of a major fast food restaurant chain.

"Each item on our menu is engineered to produce a profit."

This quote is from a presentation given by the CEO of this restaurant chain at a convention I attended in San Diego, California on February 16, 2009.

Does that sound like a company that is first and foremost concerned about the health and well being of its customers? This quote rang in my head. The thing that is most astounding about this is that the majority of our culture would not question such a statement. Why? It is because we don't clearly see the connection between food and disease.

Interestingly enough, we think that is the worst of it when, in reality, the worst of it is the hundreds of thousands of people who are ailing and dying each year because they are unknowingly consuming animal flesh that has been inaccurately labeled as nutritional and necessary food. If you don't agree that restaurants have some ownership, along with all the other food manufactures and retailers, then I strongly disagree. I think any company that sells a product should take responsibility, along with unbiased steps to test and prove the validity and safety of their products. In other words, companies in the business of food should do the necessary research on their own to realize the contribution their products make in disease creation. They should also go to whatever length is necessary to prevent the harm of others through their business. Anything short of this course of action is unconscionable. Yes, these actions should be taken even if it means shutting down a company or completely changing the course of a company's future.

When you combine these facts, it becomes obvious we do not have a resource problem; we have a thinking problem. Regardless of what you call it (ignorance, apathy, laziness, selfishness, bad habits, etc.), we have a big problem that has contributed to the entitlement culture that we current live in within our western society. Friends of mine have heard me call our land "zombieland." As a culture, we seem more interested in getting than serving, dreaming than doing, and consuming rather than assuming the responsibilities that have been bestowed upon us.

If you continue to research self-healing then you will likely come across a few unfamiliar terms. The ones below are essential to understand because of the implications they have on how our cultural perspectives have changed in terms of how we view medicine and approach healing.

Allopathic is a term originally intended to point out how traditional doctors used methods that had nothing to do with the symptoms created by the disease that meant that these methods were harmful to the patients. Early on, it was quite negative in nature, and only in the last few generations has it become acceptable by the mainstream. Generally, allopathic medicine refers to the broad category of medical practices that is sometimes called western medicine or modern medicine. The term allopathic has varying degrees of acceptance by medical professionals still today. I tend to use the term allopathic when I am talking about doctors who treat using pharmaceuticals (drugs or chemicals).

Non-allopathic would then be the opposite of allopathic. Non-allopathic medicines are also known as *naturopathic, complementary, homeopathic or alternative medicines.* Non-allopathic approaches have a much longer history than allopathic, and have only recently been displaced as the primary solutions to health-related concerns. Non-allopathic approaches have regained some ground with strong recognition in recent years, however, because they are less hazardous to our health. They actually provide some very promising results. These approaches include, but are not limited to, diet, herbs, metals, minerals, precious stones, essential oils, and non-drug-related therapies.

CHAPTER NINETEEN

Twisted Truth

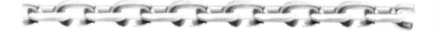

Listen closely the next time you hear a commercial for a drug. I heard one the other day, and the ad said, "Tell your doctor about <insert drug name>…" Why do we need to tell our doctor about this new drug? Because he doesn't know anything about it and the whole perspective of allopathic medicine is symptom=drug. Thus, they are simply masking the symptom and not treating the source of the problem. If you listen and act on their suggestion then you are volunteering to remain locked in your food chains.

Furthermore, do you know that doctors are restricted on what they can actually recommend for your situation based on something called standard protocol. If they recommend something outside of this then they could be putting themselves at risk of a lawsuit or losing their license to practice. Therefore, even though many doctors have learned many of the same truths that I have, they are restricted in how much of it they can share without jeopardizing their medical licenses.

Interestingly enough, I see a point in the future when pharmaceutical companies will gain the upper hand over the well-intended doctors. When you think about it, we really don't need allopathic doctors any longer. If you want to truly strip this down to what it is, simply prescribing drugs to treat symptoms, then why do we need doctors? What does the doctor generally ask you when he walks into the room? Doesn't he ask you, "What is wrong?" And are you not describing your symptoms and self-diagnosing? So what is to stop big pharmaceutical companies from lobbying for legislation that will enable them to sell their drugs directly to the consumers, via a web portal, that would enable the consumer to simply type in their symptom and have a computer tell them which drug would be best for them? It may sound far-fetched, but I would be surprised if I am the only one thinking that would be a really profitable little website.

We live in a culture that is so challenging on a day-to-day basis that we yearn for our next vacation to escape our normal existence. We no longer work for our own sustenance. Many years ago, people lived on farms and were part of a bigger community. Within the context of this community, they would gain access to all of their needs. Primarily, however, they would supply themselves with food, water, and other basics.

Today, we tend to be segmented into what we are good at, what we do, and how we make money. If we were forced to provide for all of our needs on our own, it would be impossible for most of us. I am not saying there is anything wrong with making money in various ways, and then paying someone else to do things like tilling your crops and cleaning your clothes. I am simply making the point that we live differently today then we once did.

We get up in the morning and use any number of devices throughout our day that were designed to free up our time by making life easier and more efficient. Seriously, what is it that we are working so hard to free up time for? And when is it that we actually do the thing or things that we need so desperately to create time for? If you had more time, you might write a book, read a book, spend time with family and friends in real relationship, serve the needy, start a business, do something great for your community, or maybe go on a mission trip down the block or around the globe.

I suppose the answer may be different for each of us, but I would contest that there is something more important happening as we go about our daily lives. Something that can happen in us regardless of what it is that we are actually doing. I say this because I have toiled for years attempting to earn the time to do the things I considered important. This became real to me on a trip to the ocean with my family one weekend. On this trip, one of the boxes we had planned to check on our weekend to the beach was flying a kite. Our little kids had never been in an environment where this could be done easily. This was the weekend and we had bought a couple of kites to make it happen. The problem was that one of the kites broke quickly, and the other required a much better engineer than I to get it up and keep it in the air. It was like trying to control a remote control airplane that is headed straight towards you! Which way do I turn? What do I do? Many crashes later, I began to wonder why this wasn't fun.

What I found was that I was trying to do things that others consider fun at the beach (like flying a kite) instead of doing what I value, like enjoying time with my family. For me, I needed to work on just being with my family and purposefully living out the joy that is possible for us each day. I still have a box-checking propensity, but realizing that my joy did not need to be tied to accomplishments or duties was a relief. I can go and have fun and crash kites with my kids and still feel like we had a great time just hanging out.

Living a healthy life can take some of your time. It can even take more time than eating unhealthy, but it does not have to. The first fast food appeared in the Garden of Eden. Adam and Eve would take walks for their meals, right? Along the way they would simply pluck, pick, or dig up whatever they wanted to eat at that moment. Today, it is even easier than that. We just need to walk to the kitchen, open the refrigerator door, and pick what we want. I know we actually spend more time with our food because we like to combine things to make exquisite and wonderful dishes, but the extent of what we do is our choice. My point is that if you feel like you don't have time for this, then I would challenge what your time is for, in general. What is more important than whatever you can do with loved ones over a meal? What if your meals take an average of thirty minutes more per day than they currently do, how could that bless your life?

We are surrounded by companies that are selling us products designed to make our questionable habits more efficient. We live for comfort. We will go to great lengths to protect our comfort, and that includes buying everything under the sun that we may or may not need to sustain our desire for more comfort. We protect our comfort. We worship our comfort. We even have comfort foods.

We don't actually use all the time we gain from our devices to do anything meaningful, though. In fact, we continue to buy more and more of these devices for the sake of having the latest toy. Of course we can watch five movies a week or thirteen of our favorite shows but what value does that actually bring to our lives or our surrounding world? The acquisition of the latest device is merely a status symbol. I personally think people who don't have cars are deprived. I can't imagine giving up that much freedom. But why do I think that way? Because I am programmed, thanks to our culture, to think that way. The people who choose to go without a car, an electric shaver, a ceiling fan, a microwave, or a television are not crazy. If you talk to them, they also do not feel like they are deprived. Surprise! They are getting it. They are beginning to realize their life is not about the next gadget or toy, or this or that. It isn't even about being comfortable or fully efficient. It is much greater than these.

You won't get there unless you begin to think for yourself about everything. You don't get there until you begin to question everything you are told, and the reasons for these things. And you won't get there until you put into question everything you think is real or truth. However, if you do grasp this, then you will immediately realize that you can eat whatever you want, or not. You can be whatever shape you want, or not. You can suffer and die of disease, or not. You can have a muscular stomach, or not. You can be vibrant and full of bounce and life, or not. It really is that easy. It is just a matter of saying "no" to our culture and the pervasive marketing messages, and "yes" to new thinking and a new perspective on what you do and who you are.

When we mistakenly make our lives about our food, comfort, possessions, dreams, or habits, we are bowing to false idols because we believe that idol will deliver something that it never actually will. It is a lie and the sooner we come to grips with the areas in our lives that we are believing lies, the sooner we can move on to a joyful existence!

It is more satisfying to eat less than it is to eat more. Seriously, I have done this many times. When you lay in bed with just a slight bit of hunger, you feel best and sleep best. It is a misconception that a full belly is most satisfying. In fact, in the long run it is quite the opposite. Even the short-term results are not all that enjoyable.

In fact, we have misconceptions about many things in the world around us. We're fed an enormous amount of information that, in truth, is nothing more than the attempt to manipulate our way of thinking. For instance:

…the price of an automobile doesn't actually have a lot to do with the real cost of the design and construction of the car. The actual cost is driven more by the amount the market will bear. In other words, how much the target audience is willing to pay for such a car is going to have a bigger impact on the retail cost than the amount that is spent on actually building the car. All of this is known prior to even designing the car. If they can't get the math to work out then they won't allow the project to proceed.

...milk is not good for you and it is not a good source of calcium. In fact, due to the acidic results of consuming milk, the body loses bone density.

...schools do not need more money to improve their educational performance. A big budget will bring lots of amenities and unique opportunities for the students but creative, loving energy by the instructors and a passion for learning by the students does yield much better results.

...women tend to be consistent, predictable, and relatively easy to understand as compared to their counterpart. Men are generally inconsistent, unclear, and seemingly devoid of overall mission and focus. We are duped into thinking that women are difficult to track with and understand when, in reality, it is the men that are struggling to even understand their own motivations, drives, desires, and feelings. I know from experience that I have reacted in a certain way in a given situation and then, even as it is happening, been questioning my own motives. I was first confused about understanding myself and my pride caused me to make it about others.

...separation of church and state was actually created well after the founding of the U.S. republic. Many people believe that the founding fathers of America created the idea of the separation of church and state. The truth is quite the contrary if you do a little reading. Most of the original thirteen colonies required government officials to sign an oath of trust in Jesus Christ prior to taking office.

...children beyond preschool age do not actually learn at a faster pace than adults. It seems like it when they are young because they have so much to learn to catch up with the commonly expected set of knowledge and abilities. Once they catch up with the curve, however, the learning growth tends to slow down. This is not because the capacity to learn and understand has decreased, but rather because we spend less time investing in education the older we get. Thus, we learn less and at a slower rate. A good example would be for someone that desires to learn a foreign language. They could spend months or years with a few minutes a week or they could simply travel to the appropriate geographical location and spend a month there.

Hopefully I have astounded you with at least some of the fallacies we choose to believe, or that we have been forced to believe simply due to our own ignorance and the investment of others to make sure we think a certain way. What I want you to see is that we have certain beliefs about our diet and lifestyle that act as blind spots in our thinking. Some people or companies have paid big money to lodge these assumptions into our brains. We have the full ability and right to learn the truth and to take a different path with our lives.

Do you want to be healthy? Do you want to enjoy a great body and be physically fit? Do you want to experience mental freedom like you have never had before? What is stopping you? I contest that it is nothing more than the realization that you can do whatever you want to do. Today, you can choose to ignore what you have learned about food, and begin anew with a lifestyle that will enable freedom and joy! As you do this, watch each day for the things that are not as you always thought. Take more joy in the fact that you are learning and growing as a person. This world is a dynamic environment. We think it is all about our stuff, our food, our time, and us, when, in reality, there is a whole creative and wonderful canvas that is much bigger than us.

CHAPTER TWENTY

Life On The Go

I am often asked for advice on how to be successful in making healthy choices while living a busy, on-the-go life. One of the first things that I think about is the purpose of food and making sure this is correct in our minds first.

My family doesn't get together to eat. We get together to be together, and we eat as a method of relating and enjoying time together. We don't eat first for the satisfaction of the taste or texture of the food or the pleasure that comes from it, but we eat to fuel our physical bodies so we can achieve the greater endeavors our life has been purposed for. Our purpose is not food or eating. We design and reserve space in our home for food preparation and consumption. This space, although it is designed around the food, is not first and foremost purposed for supporting eating. It is purposed for serving as an environment for life to happen. Think about a picnic table. It is designed to be sat around so that we face each other, have space for our food, and are able to focus on each other as we look across the table. If relationships were not pinnacle, then our eating environments could simply use a classroom or theater type of seating. Some of these seating arrangements are seen in some fast food establishments, but is likely designed for people who are forced to consume a meal alone. I suppose my question would be, why go to all the effort to have a meal if you can't enjoy it with someone? Is not food specifically designed to force our reliance on something external to ourselves, as well as to create a pause multiple times in our day where we naturally seek to be with each other?

I talk to many people looking for more options that support on-the-go living. Truckers are a good example, but they are no different other than they have a hyper need for more on-the-go flexibility. Truckers have it especially tough because their common stops and venues are filled with unhealthy eating options, as well as spending the majority of their time sitting. Consequently most truckers are out of shape, overweight, and generally in ill health.

I suggest truckers read to each other while they are driving. If they are alone, then there are many audio options that will enable them to continue their education. There are a number of great books that can be consumed while traveling. It may sound odd to mention this first, but continuing the education is a key component to them not giving up and just submitting to what they feel is impossible in their situation.

I then suggest that it is just as easy to stop at a grocery store like they would at a gas station or truck stop. They have large parking lots and always have produce readily available. They need to really look at more food that is in its raw, whole state. For example, they could eat cucumbers like a carrot and red peppers like an apple. This is really the best way overall, but they will want to try to get as much organic as possible because it contains fewer toxins and tastes better.

Depending upon where they are (in terms of driving), they can also have stuff either sent to them or ready for them. If they stop at home regularly, but don't stay there long, they will want to develop a home on the road within their truck.

Juicing is not impossible or too messy to do on the road or on the go. There are also some great pour-and-mix powdered products that are really helpful. This is really important, and with the right containers it is very convenient. Even if they only juice it or mix it when they stop, a ½ gallon to sip on throughout the day would be beneficial.

Because the truck is moving most of the time, I think just making the leap to eating whole raw food is going to be the best advice possible. Nuts and dried fruit is good, but can very easily become too high of a percentage of the overall intake. They are also likely not eating the nuts raw and likely don't realize that most "roasted nuts" are actually deep-fried and are therefore very unhealthy.

Burritos and various healthier packaged foods are fine as transitional food for a year or two, but ultimately they need to move away from frequent consumption of these items. They also need to be really careful to completely avoid MSG and other excitotoxins because these are very common in packaged and processed foods.

When traveling, I often do a search for a local Whole Foods or similar because I can get a great, fresh & organic salad in the deli but I can also grab some organic produce snacks, water and kombucha for my hotel room. This takes the pressure and temptation off me to eat the often-unhealthy fair served at many of the events and conventions I attend.

The biggest message all of us can take away from this is that eating "simply" is normally the very best for us and works in any situation. What I mean by eating simply is simply eating food the way it is picked off the vine, tree, or bush. A quick look, a wipe, and digestion begins! We can't get much simpler than this, and when we are living on-the-go, this is the easiest answer. The struggle is that mentally we need to make the leap to accepting the fact that a few pieces of produce can make up a meal. Once this happens, a whole new world of creativity opens up and we begin to realize the vast array of options that we have right in front of us.

I know this will be helpful as you travel about living this great life while choosing to see food as a tool rather than a reward, destination or purpose. Enjoy!

CHAPTER TWENTY ONE

Next Steps

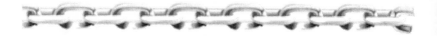

You have brains in your head. You have feet in your shoes. You can steer yourself in any direction you choose. You're on your own. And you know what you know. You are the guy who'll decide where to go.

-Dr. Seuss, *Oh, the Places You'll Go!*

As you begin this journey, let me be the first to encourage you to try to maintain focus on the things that you can and should do. If you get caught thinking about all that you are "giving up" or "can't do," you will quickly feel the sides of life folding in on you as if you are stuck, alone on a one lane road that leads to the most uninteresting, boring life you could imagine. Trust me, I can promise you from experience that although there are ups and downs along the way, I am so glad I took this path. I am more satisfied and full of life then I could ever have imagined.

I remember early on that I would literally starve myself. All I could think about were the things I normally ate, and I knew

I was not supposed to eat those things any longer. The problem was that I didn't know what to eat! I mean, I knew I could have any produce I wanted, but that can seem so uninteresting when you are making the transition. Enter transitional foods!

I ate a lot of foods along the path that were good but not great. These foods served as good transitional foods. These enabled me to get to where I am today without feeling like I had to immediately remove from my diet all the foods that I ate the first thirty years of my life. One example is making a huge burrito with all the fixings, other than meat, and enjoying it. There is value in the produce on the burrito, but it is mainly rice and beans and those are fairly neutral. This is not a lot of nutrition, but certainly progress in the right direction. There is more nutritional value than a toxic load, however. That's a good place to start. All I had to do was simply take the biggest problems (toxins) out of my food and march forward. Remember, however, that transitional foods, by the very nature of the name, should be transitional—meaning, they are temporary.

With that understanding, here are the steps I would recommend you consider as you make the transition from what is likely a fairly typical western diet to something that may seem odd at first, but with retraining you will begin to experience firsthand the vital benefits.

Although I am presenting these steps generally in chronological order, some of them may require repeated attention as you progress.

Step 1:

Increase your intake of fresh, raw, organic produce. Make this as high of a percentage of your overall intake as possible to still be comfortable with your daily living. Commit to an emphasis on greens and try not to go a day without some significant intake of green things. Begin experimenting with juicing and find some combinations you enjoy. Cut out all animal products in this step, which is anything that has a face or came from something that had a face. This includes dairy, poultry, and all other animal products. If you choose to include some transitional meat at this step, then consider one of the following seafood: salmon, flounder, sole, tilapia, or trout (according to the FDA, Office of Seafood, May 2001, these have the least amount of mercury).

Step 2:

Become a label detective. It is not necessary, but it is very likely that you will continue to eat some packaged foods. After many years, I eat very little packaged foods. However, some great snack bars, dried fruit and other items are packaged foods. These examples just happen to have clean labels (good ingredients). The major consideration at this point is avoiding all excitotoxins. You will also want to avoid refined sugars and other obviously harmful ingredients. A good rule of thumb to work towards is that if you don't understand all the ingredients, then don't buy it. I commonly look ingredients up on the Internet if I don't understand them. There are several great apps you can download to perform quick searches while shopping. You will learn a lot about various oils as you do this research and experience how you feel when you consume certain ingredients and oils. Be sure to pay close attention to how your body responds to whatever you eat. After a couple of times of not feeling well after eating something, you will often have plenty of motivation to simply choose something else.

Step 3:

Continue to Learn. This book covers the basics but it does not include your personal experience. Use this resource; mark it up and tag it as your personal handbook. The basis of step three is to continue the education while including your personal experience. Read at least two of the recommended books per year and begin to educate yourself, your family, and those around you as they have interest. If you don't have a community to lean on, then this is your opportunity to build one! Gather a group who express interest and help them. Every day we are faced with images, marketing, advertising, examples, opportunities, avenues, and habits that try to draw us down an unhealthy path. If we do not take a stand for what we know is right and true, then we stand a good chance of being courted back to the same unhealthy lifestyle that got us to the point of asking for help. We have hosted a weekly food preparation evening in our home for many years. It is an open night, and it is encouraging for us as we help and lead others. It is important that you really put down some roots in this stage. Remember the Stockdale Paradox? We must maintain a stoic belief that we will prevail in this.

Get Ready!

Don't discount the need for physical changes that may need to take place in your home, kitchen, office, workplace, or other locations. Be creative and have fun. Don't feel like you need to purchase every piece of equipment right now. The most important piece of new equipment in our home has been the VitaMix®. We use it daily, and sometimes multiple times a day. There are other helpful things like good knives, a good juicer, and a food processor, but the VitaMix® is our most utilized appliance. *Raw Food, Real World* by Matthew Kenney & Sarma Melngailis has a great list of equipment and food items to stock. It is not only a great recipe book, but a wonderful resource as well. Get a copy. Use it!

You may also begin stocking things at work to make life easier and less tempting. You may also stock or take whole food snacks (produce) with you, or maybe stash some health snack bars. These healthy convenience foods will really help you as you transition. Sometimes we trick ourselves by not doing simple things like this and then use the resulting circumstances as an excuse to not do what we know is the best for us.

For further information, bonus material, and a downloadable gift, visit:

www.foodchains.info/bonus

CHAPTER TWENTY TWO

Frequently Asked Questions

1. **What are the real problems with animal protein?**

    It is my belief that the consumption of animal products is the chief toxin that we are regularly exposed to. I also believe, based on research by Dr. Joel Fuhrman, my own research, and my personal results, the consumption of animal-sourced products causes over 90 percent of all diseases in the western culture. That is a big statement. We know that 98 percent of all medical care focuses primarily on disease-related care. I am suggesting that if we removed animal products from our diet and replaced it with a primarily plant-based diet that is free of chemicals or genetic engineering, we could nearly eliminate disease.

    Elsewhere I have given brief explanations about the problems and risks associated with animal proteins. There's not enough room or time in this book to delve any further into it. I suggest *The China Study* by Dr. T.

Colin Campbell for further information. See the recommended resources for specific info about this book.

2. **What are some good sources of protein?**

Dark, leafy greens are an excellent source of protein. The darker the greens, the better. Spinach, broccoli, kale, peas and collard are all excellent sources of protein. Although greens have the most protein per calorie, some beans, lentils and potatoes are good sources of protein as well. The bigger question here is the determination of how much protein we actually need.

3. **How much protein are we suppose to eat?**

We have three strong, healthy, beautiful children who have never had animal protein, nor do they gorge themselves on the whole foods they eat. Therefore, there must be a sufficient volume of available protein in the produce we regularly consume. See the recommended resources for information on how to get some of our family's favorite recipes.

Dr. Fuhrman answers this very question in *Eat To Live*. Here is a summary of what he believes.

The recommended daily allowance (RDA) for protein has bounced radically over the years and the metrics for protein needs have changed from animal measurements to actual human measures, which are assumed to be better or more accurate.

The World Health Organization (WHO) recommends only 5 percent of calories from protein. Even this estimate seems high to some experts. Most forms of produce contain at least 10 percent calories from protein, and green vegetables average around 50 percent.

Dr. Fuhrman recommends a high-nutrient, plant based diet which result in the intake of about 40-70 grams of protein daily. He goes on to address the question of increased need for protein due to pregnancy or of an athlete. People in these situations need a higher intake of more than just protein so an increase in overall caloric intake (more good, healthy, whole, plant based food) is required. Within a healthy regime, the additional protein will also be delivered in adequate amounts.

4. **What are some good sources of calcium?**

Dark, leafy greens are an excellent source of calcium. The bigger question here is the determination of how much calcium we actually need.

According to the recommended daily allowance guidelines (RDA), a child should consume about 200mg/day of calcium. The recommendation scale increases by age up to 1200mg/day for adults over 50. It is interesting that babies who are attempting to grow an entire new body need so much less calcium than a full grown adult who is simply maintaining a body. This assumption indicates that calcium is only used for building bones, which, of course, is false. The answer actually has more to do with our acid-forming diet than the specific growth needs of our body. A consumer of the standard western diet needs more calcium to overcome an acidic (low pH) environment in their body. In other words, westerners tend to consume a diet that causes or leaves an acidic environment in their body, which creates the need for more calcium. Calcium is a tool used by the body to neutralize acid or bring acid to a high, more alkaline state. Therefore, when we eat foods that leave an acid ash (such as meat, dairy, and sugar) our body pulls calcium from our bones to perform this necessary work. All of this leads to depletion of the bone density (or less calcium in the bones).

The big marketing lie is on the billboards with celebrities marked with a white mustache. They are advertising how good milk is for the body, and by using celebrity endorsements they're appealing to people's basic inclination to imitate those they admire. They do this knowing that when animal milk is consumed, we will need to deal with the resulting acid. They add a form of calcium to the milk, such as calcium carbonate, which can only be absorbed with sufficient resources of Vitamin D. The best source of Vitamin D is through regular sun exposure, but of course we are told we should avoid sun exposure or lather up in sunscreen, so we are generally deficient in Vitamin D as well.

On one hand the government is recommending, and even subsidizing, the meat, dairy, and egg industry so they can bring their harmful products to market at a competitive price. On the other hand, they are increasing the RDA for calcium to overcome the ill effects of these substances.

Here are some samples of good sources of calcium within a plant-based diet: seaweeds such as kelp, wakame, and hijiki; nuts and seeds such as almonds and sesame; beans; oranges; figs; quinoa; amaranth; collard greens; okra; rutabaga; broccoli; dandelion leaves; and kale.

Additionally, Dr. Fuhrman provides this chart in *Eat To Live*, showing calcium content in 100 calories of various food items:

Bok Choy 1055	Turnip greens 921
Collard greens 559	Kale 455
Romaine lettuce 257	Tofu 236
Milk 194	Broccoli 182
Sesame seeds 170	Soybeans 134
Cucumber 108	Cauliflower 88
Carrots 63	Fish 38
Eggs 32	T-bone steak 5
Pork chop 2	

The following research by others from Wikipedia further support my studies on calcium:

- Research has found an association between diets high in animal protein and increased urinary calcium loss from the bones.

- A diet high in fruit, vegetables, and cereals was demonstrated to result in greater femoral bone mineral density in older men, in comparison to a range of other diets.

- Diets high in candy were found to result in lower bone density in both men and women.

Mama was right. Eat your greens!

5. **Which juicers are better than others and why?**

First let me explain that a blender is not a juicer. Juicing is a method of separating the liquid from the fiber in living foods. There are no nutrients in the fiber. The fiber does have redeeming factors for sure, such as stimulating movement in the bowels, but the juice is the lifeblood. Blenders simply pulverize the fiber and the juice resulting in a fiber-filled, pulpy juice. There is a lot of value in blending foods because it makes the nutrients more available for absorption when they are consumed. Blending and juicing also strips the nutrients of their protective shells, so they should be consumed as quickly as possible. If they are stored, then they should be protected as much as possible from oxygen and light. A good method would be to store juice in a dark container that is filled literally to the top before being capped off. This eliminates nearly all of the oxygen that can be harmful to the nutrients.

There are generally two types of juicers available with an exception that sort of combines the two. Most industrial (designed for high volume) and low-cost juicers use a centrifugal sort of mechanism where they cut the produce into tiny pieces and then spin these pieces rapidly, thus forcing the juice from the fiber. Most low-cost juicers use the centrifugal force methodology.

The premium type of juicers is a gear-driven juicer. A gear-driven juicer is designed to grind the produce using a slow turning gear or gears that act against each other or the gear compartment. The key to these juicers is the powerful motor that enables the gears to turn slowly without slowing down or stopping. This eliminates nearly all the opportunity for heat to be generated while the produce is processed into separate juice and fiber.

The unique and fairly new type of juice that combines the two methodologies is built similar to a centrifugal juicer with the stand up spinning basket style; but instead of the high-speed spinning basket, there is a low-speed spinning auger that slowly draws the food in and presses it as it rotates. The advantage to this design is that you get a higher quality juice with easier clean up. And, the juicers are generally less expensive than their gear-driven juicer counterparts. The drawback is that I have not seen one of these type juices yet that is of really high quality. Some of them meet or exceed some of the quality standards of the centrifugal juicers but still fall short of most of the grind and press juicers.

There are generally three different designs for the gear-drive juicer to choice from, but only two of them are really realistic. The most expensive (~$2500) is called a Norwalk. The high cost and difficulty to use make it unrealistic for the average consumer. The first juicer we had was a Norwalk that was loaned to us. They are wonderful juicers in terms of the quality of juice they produce, but they are super challenging to use and clean. The method is a two-step process. The first step is inserting the produce into a shoot leading to a single slow turning gear-driven mechanism that grinds the produce into tiny bits. These bits are then gathered into a small canvas bag. This bag is then folded and placed into the second stage of the machine, which is a mechanical press. The press squeezes the fresh juice out of the tiny bits from inside the bag. The porous bag material allows the juice to flow out onto a tray and eventually into a catch basin.

We have a funny story about the first time we used the Norwalk in our kitchen. I will just say that we had carrot juice and pulp all over the kitchen, on the cabinet doors, ceiling, countertop, floors, in our hair — everywhere!

The two reasonably-priced gear-driven juicers are known as the Champion and the Green Star®, which is also called the Green Power®. The Champion has been around for the longest, and was one of the pioneer machines for bringing gear-driven technology to the marketplace. It is a single gear machine, so the produce is pushed down the throat of the machine and is mashed by a single gear. The turning action of the gear forces the mix toward the end of the machine. The juice is allowed to drain through a screen while the fiber is pushed towards the end of the machine where it exits into a catch bowl. Overall, the Champion is a good machine and can be purchased new for under $300.

The ideal juicer on the market today is the Green Star® juicer. The Green Star® is very similar to the Champion. However, it uses a twin gear design where the produce is crushed in between two slowly spinning gears. The mix is forced down the machine and a screen allows the juice to drop while the pulp continues along and out the end. The twin gear method increases the juice yield and continues the low temperature, low speed methods that are common for the gear-driven machines. A Green Star® juicer can be purchased new for under $600.

One of the big benefits of a gear-driven juicer is the ability to make nut butter and fresh fruit sorbets. Some gear-driven juicers will also allow juicing of fine greens, such as wheat grass. Although none that I know of are really good at juicing greens, there are some that have optional attachments that allow for juicing of greens. We use ours for frozen fruit sorbets regularly. When fruit begins getting over ripe, we prepare it for freezing. For example, we peel bananas and put them in bags for the freezer. Strawberries are cleaned and topped before bagging and freezing. We then pull the mix we choose from the freezer and create a sorbet (using our gear-driven juicer) or smoothie (using our Vitamix®).

Centrifugal-type juicers tend to heat the produce a bit because they are spinning so rapidly. This heat does have an impact on the quality and life expectancy of the resulting juice. Most information that I have read suggests that there is about a twenty percent to thirty percent loss in overall quality. Certainly the juice from a centrifugal type juicer is still very good quality and beneficial, especially if it is consumed soon after the juice is extracted. Centrifugal juicers made for home use usually cost significantly less than a gear-driven type juicer. Centrifugal juicers are typically $90 - $140.

My recommendation is to purchase a gear-driven juicer if you can afford it. If you want to start with a centrifugal-type juicer, then that will be fine, but plan for a 6-12 month life with regular use. During that time you look for a gear-driven juicer for less cost than retail.

Search online at websites such as eBay.com or Craigslist.org to see if you can find deals on gear-driven juicers. Stop at local garage sales or thrift stores occasionally also. Success in this would be to find a good functioning used Champion for around $100, or a Green Power® for under $200.

Since I discussed blenders in this answer, let me also recommend that you put a Vitamix® on your "to-buy" list. A good blender, such as the Vitamix®, a good juicer, a good food processor and a quality set of knives will be your kitchen staples as you learn to live and eat healthfully!

6. **Are there certain food combinations that I should be aware of that create positive or negative results?**

I don't believe it is nearly as important as some people may think to avoid certain food combinations. I am not saying that I don't think this is a valid subject. What I am saying is that it simply does not fall on the priority level anywhere near the things that someone new to this lifestyle should be considering. As you gain knowledge, this may be one of the electives that you pick up and study but, like everything as it relates to your diet, let your laboratory of one (yourself) be part of the equation in determine what works for you and what does not.

When I was diagnosed, I was encouraged to limit high-sugar foods, even raw, whole food sources such as carrot juice. To be honest, I scoffed at this. My response was something like this. "Look, if I am going to give up all this other stuff and eat what feels like a limited spectrum of foods (a mind-myth that I thankfully busted through), I am not going to concern myself with what I eat or when I eat it."

I am not advocating that this was a wise or justifiable attitude. Clearly it may not have been in my best interest. I could have followed the recommendations of the experts more closely for sure. Maybe I did, yet I just wanted a bit of control in the situation.

I think a good point to realize here is that it is easy for us to eat all kinds of fruit. Fruit is sweet and is designed to be a treat. Therefore many believe that it should only be a small fraction of the total diet.

So, to get past my less-than-optimal attitude on this subject, there are some things to learn in this area. I just don't feel like it is a starting point for someone trying to get into living a healthier lifestyle. The last thing I want for you is to finish preparing a wonderful meal, and then suddenly realize that you are eating two things that may be more difficult to digest together.

7. **Have you ever considered having someone from the medical community partner with you to formally document your story?**

We actually got to shoot a TV show with a big northwest news station a few years ago. It was a neat experience, but we were surprised that much of the show spoke of people that were failing in the methods that were considered state-of-the-art. At the same time, very little emphasis was put on the fact that we had beat melanoma and had not used the conventional medical protocol. To me, it just felt like someone needed to step back and look at the big picture of what was being shown and make some reasonable assumptions.

In terms of documenting it with a reputable medical source, I would be interested in this, but sadly, I am not sure who or what conventional medical organization would align with me. The problem for their marketing departments (yes, these are companies – medical companies with marketing budgets) is that they would not be able to draw a line to any dollars by promoting my story. Success stories are always great, but they would want the bottom line to point more people to use their modalities. In general, other than monitoring and maybe cases of partnership where people combine conventional treatments with prevention, I don't know that they would be willing to make the leap.

There may be some non-allopathic organizations that would jump at the chance, and I would enjoy those opportunities, but I am not sure that this would lead to increased validation or credibility of my story.

8. **What are your thoughts on the various methods for detoxifying?**

Our bodies are in a constant state of detoxification. We live among toxins so we have to constantly deal with this. Thankfully, we have a lot of mechanisms built into our bodies to do this work.

I know the question is more in terms of focused or intentional detoxification. I am not a big fan of detoxification diets or periods because the implication is that we are choosing to do something radical on a temporary basis to overcome long-term problems. I have heard people say that they detox one month a year, or one week a quarter, for example.

Detoxification takes months and, in some cases, years. We can choose to drop the coffee or sugar habit and only deal with the outward signs of detox for a couple of days, but the reality is that it takes weeks or months to clean our system of all of these toxins.

Our fat cells store toxins, as well, so when we make positive changes in our diet and lifestyle our bodies respond as if it is spring time! We begin to clean house. The body opens up those fat cells and begins processing the toxins that we have stored there. Sometimes this process will result in us feeling worse at certain periods because we are working through the process of removing these toxins from our system.

I am a big fan of a long-term detox approach. What that looks like is really very simple. It is a matter of providing more nutrition to our bodies on a daily basis than the toxic load we are exposed too. In other words, if we are experiencing a load of say 14 toxic buckets per day, then we would want to make sure that we counterbalance that with more than 14 buckets of nutrients. Clearly the actual measurement of these is dependant upon the severity of the toxin, or the strength of the nutrition in consideration as well as the condition of our body to effectively process the nutrients, but you get the point.

There are a couple of approaches. We can increase the amount of healthy stuff we are doing or eating, or, we can reduce the toxic load on our body where we have control over that load. Or, a little of both. The majority of the toxic load comes through the food we eat. Most of the rest comes through the air we breathe.

I have heard stories of severe detoxification. Roger's Recovery From AIDS is one of my favorite stories about detox, but I believe there is a more pleasant way of achieving the same result.

Some clinics encourage extended water fasting as a method of detox. This can be very uncomfortable and dangerous. Furthermore, it only addresses half of the problem. Water fasting eliminates most of the toxic intake, but it does not improve the nutritional side of the equation. When you look at it in these terms, you can see that fasting from toxic food and beverages is great if, at the same time, it is combined with intake of highly nutritional foods.

If the detoxification symptoms become greater than a person is comfortable with, then they can simply slow the process by eating more cooked foods. Like everything I have written, I think the focus should be on long-term success rather than short-term, 'fit-into-my-bathing-suit' results.

9. **How long should it take for food to go through my body?**

Technically, this is called "frequency." It is the transit time from the point of entry (eating) to the point of exit (defecation). It is a fairly common thought but rarely asked — by men at least!

Here is the deal. Your digestive system is a tool to provide your body with nourishment. Many people see it as an extraction tool, and it does work as that, but that isn't the primary intent. What I mean is that we see it as a machine to extract the nutrition from the things that we eat. Case in point: you eat a hamburger and think that your body will pull the nutrients from the lettuce, tomato, and ketchup, and of course the ever important protein from the meat (hopefully you know that is a myth by now), and then send it into your blood stream and throughout your body for whatever all those various organs and internal mechanisms need such things for.

Unfortunately, that is the way most of us use the digestive system. It is actually designed to quickly capture the nutrients, which are chiefly mechanically extracted with our teeth in our mouth. There is some minor chemical breakdown that happens in our stomach, but not nearly as much as we commonly burden our stomach with. In other words, the right foods provide nutrients that fit exactly with our bodies. The stomach and the rest of the system doesn't need to take a lot of action to extract the nutrition.

I will use myself as an example since my body has been a well-analyzed, living laboratory for many years.

I head to the bathroom every time I eat but most especially in the morning about 30 minutes after I eat or drink something. It is a natural reaction for your body to clean out the old and make space for the new. The actual transit time (time it takes to pass through) should be well less than 24 hours. Any guess what the typical transit time is for a westerner's diet? The average study reports about seventy-two hours. Here is something else to think about. What happens to a bunch of fresh raw produce if you put it in the blender, and then let it sit out at room temperature for twenty-four hours? Not much right? In fact, it will definitely still contain some life. Now think about the burger. If you blend that up (you will naturally have to add some soda pop so it will blend properly in the blender, right?) and set it out on the counter at room temperature for three or four days, what is it going to look and smell like?

The problem is that certain foods make your digestive system sluggish and it does not push as aggressively as it normally would. This is caused primarily with low-fiber foods. Did you know that animal products do not contain a bit of fiber? Fiber is what activates the contractions within your intestines; it keeps things moving on through. Produce is all fiber, other than the water that is packed with the essential nutrients. The nutrient-packed water is the life-blood of the plant and our bodies. The fiber is just the carrier, so wouldn't it make sense that it would cause your intestine to contract and push it through?

The intestine is designed to be a one-way tool. Once the food passes a certain point, toxins and additional water should be added to the intestines, but nothing should be coming the other direction. Everything should be on a one-way train to the light at the end of the tunnel. What happens when food lingers in the digestive track is that it builds up a high level of toxins, which are then able to work their way back into our system.

So, how do you increase the trips to the outhouse? Eat more fiber! It will stimulate your intestines and encourage the movement of much of the muck and pus that builds up from tons of carbohydrates and animal protein. Talk about an easy way to drop a few pounds quickly! Just increase your intake of raw, plant-based foods. There are also some herbs that can help stimulate the bowels into action. If you persist in eating a western diet then you may consider a periodic cleanse with something like this. I am not saying it is good to eat like our culture does, but the idea of all those toxins building up inside is a definite problem for western-diet eaters.

Since we are in this region, some of you may know of or wondered about rectal itching. It is caused by parasites (more toxins) escaping (being forced out) during the natural detox process. It isn't supposed to last long, but can be expected if you make some improvements in your eating habits as your body begins to cleanse.

10. **What does the term "organic" really mean, and who polices the use of this?**

Organic, to me, means that food is grown based on the original intent. For example, a seed is put in the ground, watered, and allowed sunlight until it produces a result such as fruit. The technical term, 'organically grown,' means that this process must be free of fertilizer, other chemicals, or additives in the soil or during the growing process.

I will get back to my definition in a moment, but for now, let's look at the perspective of other sources. The diversity of opinions or applications of definitions is interesting, maybe even a bit scary. This information may cause you to question the use of the term "organic" all together. Hopefully, in the end, these facts will force us to realize that everything comes down to the basis for truth that each of us uses. If that basis varies, then the results will equally vary. Where there is no apparent basis for truth, we find people who make decisions based on self-serving factors. These people live completely devoid of the natural conscious responsibility that a person, who understands foundational truth, demonstrates.

Dictionary.com has several definitions for "organic." Definition number nine states: "Developing in a manner analogous to the natural growth and evolution characteristic of living organisms; arising as a natural outgrowth."

This is a fancy way of saying what I said. I agree with this definition.

Definition number eleven from dictionary .com says, "Pertaining to, involving, or grown with fertilizers or pesticides of animal or vegetable origin, as distinguished from manufactured chemicals."

Basically, what it says is that we can and should call something 'organic' provided that whatever we use as fertilizers or pesticides comes from a plant or an animal. This is not initially shocking but the implications are tremendous. Basically, what it says is that it is okay to label something 'organic' provided that the ingredients used to accelerate growth are from so-called natural (plants and animal) sources. What bothers me is that we could so easily include animal substances in this mix. Little do most of us know that one of the most-used substances from an animal for fertilizing is excrement. Looking just at the economics, this is a very reasonable way of getting growth encouragers (such as nitrogen, phosphorus and potassium) into the soil. There are a number of negative effects of this, but without belaboring this any longer, I just want to make the point that we can actually grow great produce without using animal products for fertilizing or as a pesticide.

From Wikipedia under the heading "Organic Food":

Organic foods are made according to certain production standards. For the vast majority of human history, agriculture can be described as organic; only during the 20th century was a large supply of new synthetic chemicals introduced to the food supply. This more recent style of production is referred to as 'conventional,' though organic production has been the convention for a much greater period of time. Under organic production, the use of conventional non-organic pesticides, insecticides, and herbicides is greatly restricted and saved as a last resort. However, contrary to popular belief, certain non-organic fertilizers are still used. If livestock are involved, they must be reared without the routine use of antibiotics and without the use of growth hormones, and generally fed a healthy diet. In most countries, organic produce may not be genetically modified. It has been suggested that the application of nanotechnology to food and agriculture is a further technology that needs to be excluded from certified organic food. The Soil Association (UK) has been the first organic certifier to implement a nano-exclusion.

The inclusion of this from Wikipedia leaves more questions than it provides answers on, but I felt that including it here would help lay the foundation for how really vague the definition of organic really is. Furthermore, I wanted to show how daunting it would be to manage the implementation of the standard related to growing something organically. The main point that I would like to expand upon is the idea that the modern use of the term, 'organic,' is something new. The Wikipedia text makes it clear that organic is much more common and historical than the new conventional methods of chemically affecting the crops and soil.

I will close my definition phase here with another quote from Wikepedia. I think this is interesting because it shows the five general guidelines or requirements for becoming organically certified.

From Wikipedia under the heading "Organic Certification":

Organic certification is a certification process for producers of organic food and other organic agricultural products. In general, any business directly involved in food production can be certified, including seed suppliers, farmers, food processors, retailers and restaurants. Requirements vary from country to country, and generally involve a set of production standards for growing, storage, processing, packaging and shipping that include:

- *avoidance of most synthetic chemical inputs (e.g. fertilizer, pesticides, antibiotics, food additives, etc), genetically modified organisms, irradiation, and the use of sewage sludge;*

- *use of farmland that has been free from chemicals for a number of years (often, three or more);*

- *keeping detailed written production and sales records (audit trail);*

- *maintaining strict physical separation of organic products from non-certified products;*

- *undergoing periodic on-site inspections.*

In some countries, the government oversees certification, and commercial use of the term organic is legally restricted. Certified organic producers are also subject to the same agricultural, food safety and other government regulations that apply to non-certified producers.

In my definition, I describe a perfect world sort of scenario. We put a seed in the ground, the rain waters it, the sun shines upon it and after a certain amount of time we harvest fruit. But because we cannot trust all farmers to adhere to such growing practices out of philosophical convictions, we have to create intense certification standards.

One of the big things we need to understand as it relates to organic farming is, what I call, "factory farming." Until recently, most produce was grown on small family-like farms. It was more of a garden-like environment. Farmers found that specific plant varieties and planting techniques deterred pests and increased the yield. They also learned that picking the produce at a certain time of the day reduced the amount of bugs being captured within the produce. Ultimately, these families may have gone on a walk for most of their meals, quite literally eating as they worked. Regular, sit-down meal preparation may have been an occasion rather than commonplace.

Fast-forward to today, with miles of land skimmed flat and tilled, turned, planted, watered and harvested by machines. Of course in this factory farm we need a mechanism to protect the crops. The corn and peas really enjoyed growing together on the family farm and provided each other necessary protections; but today, within thousands of acres of corn, there are no peas in sight. So we need to introduce some chemicals to protect the corn from the bugs. While we are at it, why not also include some additional chemicals that will help the plants grow more rapidly? After all, if I can turn the crop more quickly (similar to manufacturing turns in a factory), then I can yield a better result for the shareholders (it is all about money).

I lightly covered the part of the question having to do with regulation of the established standards. Given the length of my answer already, I will limit my response here and just encourage you to read up on the role the United States Department of Agriculture (USDA) plays in managing the organic standards within the U.S. and the International Federation of Organic Agriculture Movements (IFOAM) for international information.

11. **What can I do to repair a chronic kidney problem?**

See my answer to Question 13 below. I have a friend who had a chronic kidney problem, which he was told was incurable by his doctors. He started juicing and eating greens, and over an 18-month period he lost about 200 pounds and cured his kidney problem as well as a long list of other ailments. Question everything. Just because someone says something is impossible doesn't mean that it actually is really, truly impossible. It likely means that either they don't know the way, or they don't have the energy to make it happen.

12. **What can I do if I have had a surgery that has removed an organ such as my thyroid?**

This is a great question. I don't have any in-depth answers because I think I would get into the zone of prescribing if I did. My intention is to educate and illuminate, not to prescribe or direct. If we get a part of our body removed, in many cases, the rest of the body has mechanisms to be able to overcome these situations. Certainly if someone has their heart or brain removed, then that would pose a rather difficult dilemma, but other, less critical organs or parts can often be overcome.

What is most important in these situations, and in the point of any diagnosis, is that we do not lose hope. The greatest hope that I know is in choosing to live as healthy as possible given the choices that we have at our fingertips, and to avoid as much toxicity as possible. Beyond that, we do not have any control. However, because we do not have ultimate control, does that give us license to ignore what we can do? I think not. I encourage everyone, in every circumstance, to do all they can and leave the rest to our Maker. At times, it is going to feel like we do a lot of the work, and at other times we are going to realize that we do very little of what needs to be done. Also, at times, we are going to experience loss due to someone being taken by disease or illness.

I know someone who came to some of our classes that had a very serious cancer diagnosis. He looked in very tough shape from the day that I met him and I doubted his ability to win his fight. Nevertheless, considering his circumstances, he was employing everything conventional medicine technique. He eventually lost the battle, but he did so peacefully and without a tremendous amount of pain. I don't know if the cancer had just spread too far or if the modalities of the medical treatment he was also utilizing were the cause. I also do not know the extent to which he really adopted what I did.

13. **Are there certain types of produce that help overcome disease?**

All of them! Let me share with you my perspective on the problems with our health care system as it does actually relate to this question. One of the main problems is that we call healthcare, well, "healthcare." It isn't health-care at all. Dr. Tel Oren recently said in a seminar that 98 percent of the energy expelled within the hospitals and clinics of the western world is done combating disease. Should we not call this "disease care" instead? After all, we are working on attempting to fix disease, right? Where does disease come from? Disease comes directly through, and from, the lifestyle choices that we make each and every day as we walk through our lives.

If you want cancer, then a recipe is readily available for you. If you would like heart disease, diabetes, or multiple sclerosis, then step right up and pick up a recipe. We know how to create each of these. Why then is it so difficult to reverse-engineer our actions to the point where we accept and understand that we are quite literally creating these diseases within our own bodies? The problem with that is everyone would be forced to accept the fact that nearly all physical health conditions are a result of their own actions. That is like saying a dirty word in church. Don't tell people what they are doing wrong or they might feel bad. That would just be politically incorrect.

Instead, let's tell the people that they need more doctors and pills so they can feel well again. Let's burden the entrepreneurs and their companies with the responsibility of balancing an impossible budget by demanding health insurance that is laden with high costs as a direct result of poor lifestyle choices.

We need to take a systematic approach to health care. It needs to begin with the understanding that there are three separate elements to the care. The first is disease. The second is accident, and the third is prevention.

These are the three pillars that our health care system should be built upon. Accident care represents less than two percent of the overall expenditure of the system. Thankfully, we have great hospitals, doctors, and drugs to help us through times of serious trauma. Yes, I did just say that! Remember, I am a racecar driver. I enjoy the comfort of knowing that emergency rooms today have the capabilities to deal with such things. I don't want any of that to change. I just want us to look at it differently.

Prevention needs to take center stage. It is going to happen first and foremost through good education. This is teaching that emphasizes the power that we have in our choices about our food and our lifestyles. This will lead to a revolution of sorts where we will force the suppliers of our food to give us what is healthy, in addition to what they can make a profit on, instead of just the latter.

This sort of approach will also prevent the bloated bureaucracy of Washington D.C. from forcing businesses to pay for disease care they simply can't afford. If that does happen, then it would be the undoing of the entire entrepreneurial system that built this country, because there would no longer be any motivation to build or grow. Why? Because the precedence would be such that the government would simply take anything that we earned. Furthermore, the people would feel the backlash of such a decision because they would quickly learn that the small businesses they work for cannot afford the disease care coverage the government is requiring, and will either respond by lowering wages or closing the doors. Either way, the people lose. We need to step back and work for long-term sustainable results and stop looking for momentary gain.

So, what would I eat if I had a disease? Well, I do have a disease. I have lots of them. One is cancer, and what I do for that is I eat lots of raw, fresh, organic produce. Is there certain produce that brings about better results? Yes! The best, most nutrient-dense foods on the planet are dark, leafy greens of all sorts and kinds. I eat them and enjoy them in abundance. Second to that, I am not sure the mix of food I eat has a big impact. I primarily eat what looks, smells, and tastes good, provided it is in a whole food state.

14. What role do you feel exercise has in a healthy life?

Other than an active lifestyle over the first 10+ years I have been eating healthy, I didn't have a good understanding of exercise. Unsurprisingly, I also did not have a plan for regular exercise. I have always been fairly active, which helped, but not active enough in my view to really achieve the physical results that I wanted. And, thankfully, 20 minutes in the kitchen does save 3 hours in the gym. So, because I was doing so well in the kitchen I was experiencing weight loss and some level of fitness. But, just like my food chains, I was equipped with some hardy exercise chains as well! I thought that being athletic meant I had to be at the gym for what looked like a 1-2 hour cycle several times a week. Because of this thinking, I never exercised significantly because I simply didn't feel I had the time.

Then, one day, I read, *Great By Choice*, a business-focused book written by a favorite author of mine, Jim Collins. This particular publication was not nearly has helpful to me in my professional work as it was with my thinking on exercise, however. In fact, the story of the 20-Mile-March pretty much knocked me over with regards to my perspective on exercise.

In summary, the 20-Mile March is about two separate expeditions happening at the same time to the South Pole. These would be the first groups to ever reach the South Pole. One group was lead by a man who resolutely led in completing 20 miles a day regardless of weather conditions. The second group only traveled as far as they wanted on nice days but would stay in their tents when conditions were difficult for hiking.

In the end the first group beat the second group by several weeks. However, the reason for the second group's failure was that they ran out of provisions and all perished on the return after the discouraging realization that they had lost the race to the South Pole.

This simple little story got me to thinking about exercise and helped me to realize that I had to question some things about my perspective on exercise. I began to question my thinking that exercise required an hour of my day every day. No longer bound by an hour mandate, I considered what length of time would I complete every day without fail. I landed on 5 minutes a day, so I designed a simple body weight and cardio routine using some very common exercises. I practiced this routine eleven consecutive months, only missing about one day a month. This effort and the resulting physical improvements led me to question if I even had more than 5 minutes a day that I wanted to invest.

It has been more than 2 years since I started this exercise plan. I released a book called, *The 5-Minute Workout* in 2013 to help others implement this adaptable exercise routine into their own lives.

15. **I have heard you say that drugs don't cure. If they don't, then what do they do? And how do I achieve healing or cure without them?**

There is no drug on the planet that cured anything, nor has there ever been to my knowledge. That may be difficult to believe, considering how much we are taught to trust in those colorful pills, but it is true. The effect of drugs is simply to change the symptoms that we experience.

Isn't it interesting that we see an ad for a drug, happy and positive, and then we turn the page only to see a fine printed page full of all the side effects? What are these side effects? Well, they are actually the primary effect of the drug. Among these primary effects is a masking of your symptoms if you are one of the unlucky ones.

Does that sound backwards? It should. The unlucky get their symptoms masked by a drug so they keep taking the drug forever. If they were cured, would they not stop taking the drug and go on about their lives? That is why they are unlucky, because they stop looking for the cure.

If they got to the end of their rope, with no possible drug in sight to cure, then maybe they would attempt some alternative methods such as changing the way they eat. This is again another interesting use of words. Why do we call anything, outside of conventional medical treatments that have only been around for a few decades, alternative methods? We do that because we are copying the marketers, and that is the way they speak. The reality is that many of the natural methods, especially dietary and lifestyle choices, are much more common and have more history than any of the conventional treatments.

The only way we can achieve healing or a cure is through the work of our own individual body. Our self-healing mechanisms need to do the work required to achieve healing on a daily basis. If those mechanisms are compromised or weak, then they are going to slowly lose the battle. The best we can do is to strengthen our self-healing systems so that we maintain a healthy physical state at all times.

16. What were the first indications that you were successful with your diet changes?

Within a few days, I felt much better than I had in years. I began sleeping better almost instantly, and I felt some of the mind fog lift in just a few days. My skin tightened, I had hope, and I just felt good. I am still amazed at how resilient our physical bodies are. We can abuse them for decades, and then after only a few days of eating healthy, we can receive some amazing results.

17. What is the difference between consuming animal flesh and fish?

Dr. Campbell, in *The China Study*, covers the problems with animal protein in good detail. He also presents the information in a way that is easily understood and motivational. The position from Dr. Campbell and other professionals and individuals, is that the animal protein actually causes many of the physical problems that we experience. I have yet to read anyone who includes fish in the same category, however, because fish protein is structurally different from other animal protein. The main concern with fish is that many of the fish species contain a high amount of heavy metals and even radiation that is toxic to our bodies. Mercury is specifically discussed because it is found in many different types of sea life.

18. Explain GMO.

According to Wikipedia, a genetically modified organism (GMO), or genetically engineered organism (GEO), is an organism whose genetic material has been altered using genetic engineering techniques. These techniques, generally known as recombinant DNA technology, use DNA molecules from different sources, which are combined into one molecule to create a new set of genes. This DNA is then transferred into an organism, giving it modified or novel genes.

For example, this technology has been used to create a "terminator gene" within certain crops. Corn is one that has experienced heavy genetic engineering. The terminator gene was designed to create infertile crops. In other words, the seeds would yield one cycle, but if the farmer attempted to plant the terminator-infected seeds, they would not grow. Why would anyone do this? The reason is that the companies can put a patent on the seed (or at least attempt to), and thus take ownership of a particular crop seed or version of the seed. In doing so, they force the growers to return year after year to buy their seeds.

As if this technology wasn't bad enough, you may have noticed that I talk about this in the past tense. The reason is that the terminator gene presented some serious social problems if it somehow spread or infested other non-GMO seeds—which, of course, it did. So, how did they respond? They designed another type of impotent seed. This one will grow normally and will reproduce in subsequent years, but only if the farmer purchases the proper fertilizer. This magic mix comes, of course, from the same company trying to dominate the seed market in the first place. Now, they don't actually have to manage the seed stock any longer. The farmers will do it for them, and return year after year to purchase the magic mix to make the seeds grow.

You vote in the way you spend your money. I urge you to demand non-GMO products in all your purchases. The implications of GMO are limitless and discomforting.

19. What is wrong with soy products?

The biggest problem with soy products is they are nearly all GMO. Tofu, a common soy product, represents only part of the greater bean or edamame (soy). Tofu is made by coagulating the juice from soy beans. This is done using various different methods, but is questionable secondarily to the fact that it initially came from a GMO source, because it is no longer a whole food and requires significant processing to produce.

There are lots of options to every soy product, and therefore I see no reason to take any risk by regular consumption of soy or soy products.

20. Can you explain water quality? It seems like there are so many options and I am confused.

I have been asked by several people to represent or endorse their water machines the last couple of years. The main push is in the area of water ionizer machines. These machines are fascinating. They can literally change the state of plain water and make a highly alkaline water that has some benefits to our bodies (because those eating the standard western diet tend to be acidic), or turn the same water into an acid strong enough to sterilize.

The problem with the ionic machines is that they don't perform the same function as a distillation process, which is to remove the toxins. Distilling is not perfect either, because it also removes the necessary minerals that exist in the water. Drinking only distilled water for long-term can actually leech our bodies' resources rather than fill them. If you are using distilled water, the latest recommendation includes adding some sort of liquid mineral back to the water after distilling.

With the best technology that we have today, it seems that the following process (in this order) would yield the most ideal water, other than water directly from a plant:

- Distillation

- Ionization
- Add living minerals back

The problem is that the equipment for achieving the above is not readily available. It could be easily built, but it just has not been done yet.

Remember that the absolute ultimate best water on the planet for our consumption is found inside living produce. Something magical happens during the photosynthesis process. The result is a living water found only within a living plant. That is where the nutritional value comes from with our consumption of produce. The produce is made up of fiber and water. The fiber is simply a carrier for the nutrients, and the nutrition is found in the water. Don't be fooled into believing that you need a certain amount of plain drinking water everyday. The more raw, whole foods you eat, the less necessary supplementing with drinking water is.

21. **Why is it that many vegetarians are just as unhealthy as non-vegetarians? That fact deters me from even trying a vegan or vegetarian diet.**

You may come across "social vegans" at some point. Nikki and I visited a vegan pub recently for fun. My guess is that the proprietors created the establishment mainly out of concern for animals. Nearly all of the menu items were deep-fried. Social vegans do not generally eat for their health but instead they simply want to avoid eating animal products. The result is a diet that is laden in processed foods and empty calories. They remove the toxins, but they do not load the system with highly nutritional foods that are low in calories.

The other reason that we see vegetarians in poor physical state is chiefly due to the fact that most vegetarians continue to eat dairy products. Dairy contains a concentration of animal protein and is therefore just as harmful, if not more so, than an actual steak.

CHAPTER TWENTY THREE

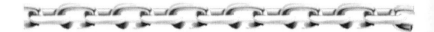

Q&A –Nikki Sessler

1) **How did you feel when Jerrod was diagnosed with metastasized cancer?**

I was totally devastated. We had just been married two years, had both quit our jobs in the past six months, our insurance did not cover us in this case, and we were hoping to start our family. After the initial shock of it all, I did find peace in knowing God had a plan for our lives and that this must somehow play into that. At the time, neither Jerrod nor I had any idea of how that would be. However, God has continually and amazingly opened the doors for our story to be shared.

2) **What has been your greatest struggle with this diet and lifestyle change?**

First a little history on how I grew up eating. It was just my mom and me living at home during my childhood. I never thought about it at the time, but she didn't like fruit or vegetables. We never had any in the house, not that I would have eaten them then even if we had. With that said, my diet consisted of hamburgers, pizza, soda, and candy bars. The only salad we ever had was something my mom would make with a big piece of iceberg lettuce laid on a plate, a banana sliced in half on top of it, topped with mayonnaise and walnuts. Until I met Jerrod, I had never had many different vegetables, including broccoli or asparagus. My greatest struggle with this diet and lifestyle choice is dealing with an addiction I have to soda and not giving into the cravings I have for the food that I grew up with, even though I know how bad they are. It is also a struggle knowing that people look up to me, because I am married to Jerrod. I don't feel like I should be looked up to because I'm dealing with these other issues. It makes me feel hypocritical sometimes. I believe 100 percent in this program and what a difference it can make. I just feel badly I don't always live the example for people to follow.

Another particularly difficult challenge for me was taking the BarleyMax® nutritional supplement. I had a hard time with that. When I was using the capsules, it wasn't difficult at all, because I couldn't taste it. However, mixing the powder with liquid and drinking it is a better way to absorb it, so I switched to this less-palatable form. I also struggled with consuming a high percentage of raw food, and eating most of that in vegetables. Our family, like most in our culture, has propensity towards cooked food. A little is fine, but it can easily become more than we really want it to be. We do a lot of salads, but even in our salads we use tomatoes, cucumbers, avocados, and bell peppers, which are technically all fruits (Hallelujah Acres recommends the majority of the 85 percent raw be vegetables vs. fruits).

Jerrod: Nikki is wonderful and I am so proud of her for what she has done in terms of diet and lifestyle choices for our family and herself. I try to remind her that she has made it seventy percent of the way from where she was rather than her tendency to focus on the distance she still has to travel. Possibly like you, Nikki wasn't facing a terminal illness like I was when she began this journey. I was. I often tell people that the choices on a day-to-day basis were not as difficult for me as they will be for those who choose it by conviction instead of necessity. You see, every time I lifted my fork, I thought one of these two words, "life" or "death." I knew that if I chose "death" too many times it was going to be the result for me. I am proud of Nikki for making these tough but rewarding changes!

3) **As Jerrod's wife, what challenges have you faced to try to accommodate his dietary desires?**

Jerrod likes a variety when it comes to his food. For instance, when we make salads, he will sometimes open the spice drawer and just start pouring different spices into his salad. This is not my style. I have not always been overly comfortable in the kitchen. I did not spend any time there while I was growing up, and I don't always feel like I do a good job when I am there. Thankfully, I have had many years of practice and instruction from taking a raw chef certification course. Taking this course with our daughter, Farrell, has really helped me gain confidence in the kitchen. However, I sometimes still use recipes and do not stray far from the instructions.

4) **What would you say to someone who is considering this diet in light of facing serious physical problems?**

Do it! What do you have to lose? There are so many testimonies of how this program has turned people's lives around from death's door. Our own family has examples of how we've benefited from this in the drastic changes that occurred. As a trial before really committing to this lifestyle, our entire family (moms, brothers, and sisters) did it with us. We were seeing if it really worked. My mom, who is diabetic and has a list of other health issues, was one of our co-pioneers. In three months, she lost six dress sizes, was off her high blood pressure medicine, and almost completely off of her diabetes medicine. Unfortunately, she didn't want to make the permanent change and chose not to continue. She quickly gained all of the weight back, plus some. As she ailed from her diseases, she had to have all of the toes on her right foot and eventually most of her foot amputated because of diabetes. I sure wish she would have stayed on the program. Even if your situation is terminal it still makes more sense to adopt a healthy lifestyle. The last thing you want to do in these situations is contribute to an already unhealthy environment. You may not be perfect but that is ok.

5)   **What was the pregnancy process like without animal products?**
I didn't find it difficult going without animal products during my three pregnancies. The hardest part was dealing with midwives, doctors, concerned friends, and family who didn't understand why we've made the choice not to include that in our diet. All three of our kids have been very healthy since birth and have never had any animal products.

6)   **What special accommodations have you adopted in order to raise kids in a culture contrary to your family's lifestyle?**
We bring our own food with us pretty much everywhere we go. When we travel, we have a cooler full of food for us to eat. When we fly, we stop at a supermarket and go shopping to load up our hotel room. When we go out, we are very selective and make sure the places we go are accommodating to our needs. We have had great luck with Mexican, Thai, and soup & salad restaurants (as long as we make sure they don't use MSG). Our kids are often invited to friends' houses for parties or play dates. I make sure we bring

our lunch or our own treats. For the birthday parties, we are always asked, "What do you do about the birthday cake?" Our kids love fruit leathers, snack bars, and other healthy treats they don't get at home very often. When we go to parties, I bring those along for them to have instead of cake. They have not once asked to have cake instead of their treats. At the last party we went to, a friend of Gabe's (our oldest) asked if he could have what Gabe was having instead of the cake. Lucky for him I brought extra!

7) **When talking with people who are facing a difficult physical ailment, what do you recommend as first action steps?**

First, wrap everything in prayer. Second, stop eating meat and dairy products, start drinking fresh juices, and begin eating a lot of salads.

Jerrod: I would suggest a strong approach to self-education as well. There are many times when my willpower failed, but the knowledge came through to assist me in doing what was right.

8) **What do you think your life would look like if you had not learned about this healthy lifestyle?**

From the diagnoses the doctors were giving us, I know we wouldn't have three gifts from God that we have right now (Gabe, Farrell, and Jake). I also think it is very likely I would have been a widow at a young age. I am so thankful and grateful to Jerrod's Uncle Brad and Aunt Patti for introducing us to this lifestyle, but also to the hundreds of people along the way that have encouraged us an allowed and spoken into our lives.

9) **What is it like being married to an engineer-turned entrepreneur who likes to drive racecars?**

It is very exciting, but at the same time very stressful. Jerrod is great at what he does on and off the track, but that doesn't help the knot my stomach gets into when he gets in the car.

10) What is your favorite food?

I love to snack on tomatoes, cucumbers, nuts, and homemade guacamole. We also enjoy having cheese-less pizza every now and then as a treat.

Raising Healthy Kids

Since Nikki was willing to share in this section, I thought it would also be good to talk about raising healthy kids. We have a ton to learn in this area but we have gained much wisdom from experience. Some has been just good basic common sense and some has been from others.

Immunizations

Immunization is a delicate and often stress-filled subject, mostly because of all the cultural pressure to stay within the typical social lines. It seems nearly every month now we are hearing a story of an otherwise well-meaning family being torn apart because of their unwillingness to submit to conventional medical treatments. Granted, some of these stories are a bit extreme, and clearly these people are completely ignorant and misled in terms of true nutrition. The reality is that Nikki and I are lumped into the same category by the population, and more importantly by the courts of the land. If one of our kids were to fall ill, for example, to the swine flu, and it was found out that we refused immunizations, then we could quickly find ourselves facing jail time or worse—being forced to subject our family's bodies to deadly toxins.

Needless to say, this has been a topic of discussion and prayer within our home for many years. In many ways, we would prefer no one knew we refused immunizations. However, we also know we must lead with the truth. I realize some risk of backlash comes from this. I also realize that for many people a blanket disregard for immunizations is possibly not the correct option. If, for example, a family is not going to commit to a healthy diet and they plan to continue to consume foods and toxins that deflate the immune system from performing at the very highest level, then some immunizations may be best. For some, it is conceivable they may benefit from the "drugs" called immunizations. Others may be permanently affected or even die because of the toxic load.

Pregnancy

The ability to achieve a healthy pregnancy is becoming more challenging and seems impossible for some. We have first-hand experience with several couples that have had success getting pregnant once they got their diet in line to balance their systems. It is an honor to know that some children are now alive, in part, because their parents learned the truth about the impact of diet and lifestyle on their ability to be successful in pregnancy.

In my mind, I see a sort of mineral storehouse inside our bodies. In this storehouse there exist slots with labels for all the various vitamins, minerals, hormones, and such that our bodies need to function on a day-to-day basis. After all, it takes a lot of work to make hundreds of thousands of new cells to replace the dying ones each day. It needs some raw materials. Picture each of those ice tray slots with a different label for a certain nutrient we need. If your diet is deficient in certain items, then that slot will stay empty for a long time. This will cause, in some cases, big problems within the body.

Here is one example: anytime we consume an acidic food (a food that creates or leaves an acid ash within our system may not necessarily have an extremely low pH when it enters the digestive system), our bodies must balance the ash to keep our overall pH within a safe range. One of the mechanisms for accomplishing this is by neutralizing acid with calcium. If the nutrient storehouse is low on calcium then the bones serve as a good resource for calcium. Thus, our system will borrow some calcium from the bones. Over a long period of time, this creates a disease called osteoporosis (weakened bones), which is a loss of the calcium that once provided bone density.

My mom suffered from osteoporosis for years prior to making significant diet changes. She has now been able to return her bone density back to the normal range. What happened? When she began to eat right, her nutrient storehouse was filled up, and she was able to begin paying back the bones for the calcium she had borrowed over the years.

Interestingly enough, dairy contains animal protein, which leaves an acid ash. One of the big chants we hear for the promotion of dairy is that it contains supplemental calcium. The reality is that we need calcium to attempt to overcome the negative effects of an unhealthy, acid diet, which is chiefly driven by the consumption of animal products. It seems to make sense to me that we can simply stop eating the things that cause or leave an acid ash, then we can stop the massive supplementation in an attempt to balance an unhealthy system.

The point with this as it relates to pregnancy is that it could be that there is a mismatch in the necessary nutrients to either build a baby, or to even conceive. If your body is not fit to build a healthy baby then it may have some precautionary measure to prevent pregnancy from even happening. This is just theoretical, of course; but either way, the result is the same and filling up the nutrient storehouse provides the best opportunity.

We have been through three fairly uneventful pregnancies. Well, pretty uneventful for me, that is. Nikki has a few words for me when I try to diminish her challenges of pregnancy. What I mean is that it seems like they were pretty much in alignment with about the smoothest possible pregnancies that one could have. Conception, when desired or attempted, was never a problem. Our kids are all pretty close to two years apart. Nikki supplemented with folic acid, B12, and a good prenatal vitamin just to be safe during each of the pregnancies. Our diet has continued to improve over the years, so Gabe, our oldest, would have gotten the muddiest ride in terms of Nikki's nutritional storehouse and ability, but he seems to be doing just fine. Nikki remains free of stretch marks of any kind.

We did keep up with regular doctor visits during the pregnancy with Gabe, but we also met with our doula (experienced woman who assists before, during, and after childbirth) regularly because she understood our lifestyle perspective. She walked us through the pregnancy and birthing process, teaching us along the way. This turned out to be a life-saver for us once the birthing began. With Farrell and Jake, we used a midwife and the same doula, so the regular visits were in a much more comfortable environment with people who really understood, appreciated, and agreed with our naturalistic approach to pregnancy.

The final trimester of each pregnancy is always the most memorable, especially the last month. For Gabe, we were not nearly as impatient, but for Farrell and then Jake, the last month seemed like an eternity. Nikki wanted the baby out and I just wanted whatever she wanted!

We greatly miss the child of one pregnancy that started unplanned and ended the same. We have always been excited about having a big family, and so even though a fourth pregnancy was a surprise, it was a welcome one. About three months into it, we made a trip, as a family, on an airplane to attend a wedding. Had we known how that flight would impact the pregnancy, we certainly would not have taken it. During the visit, we lost the baby. We will never forget that trip. Nikki was in emotional pain immediately, but for some reason I tried to shrug it off. A few months had to pass before I really hurt for the situation. I hurt because I love each of our kids so much that I wonder what another would have been like. Their personalities are so different from each other, and I feel that we lost something so precious that we can't even fathom it. Nothing can or replace that baby. I love kids and I hope we have more, but I will always have a special spot for the one we lost.

Birth
All of our kids were in the neighborhood of six pounds at birth. I remember as a kid that many of us were five or six

pounds, and it was totally odd that we would hear of any newborn being more than eight pounds. That is the reason why I find it so interesting today that people think nothing of the fact that babies have gotten so much bigger. Is it just me or is it really obvious that the size of the baby has a direct relationship with the eating habits of the mom? I blame dairy products first, but I know that there are a lot of other contributing factors. Just plain overeating is a problem as well. Dairy is designed to take a relatively small calf, and make it into a full-grown animal of hundreds of pounds. Clearly there is too much fat and too much of the wrong type of protein in it for it to be of any use to us as humans.

Gabe was born in a big regional hospital. He was carried full term, and the day the water broke our doula was there in a flash to help us. We stayed at home for the first few hours until we transitioned to the hospital. We opted against all drugs and monitoring equipment. Doctors checked the dilation when we arrived and infrequently thereafter. Nikki was moving along well, but there was a problem that would halt progress for several hours. As Gabe's elongated head crowned, the problem was clear. The umbilical cord was wrapped around his neck, holding him back. After it was pulled over the top of his head, he popped right out.

The biggest challenges we faced with the birthing process was the disrespect from the medical staff toward our birthing plan. I was also amazed at the ambivalence of the doctor attending and the actual birth. I realize that this may have been her 10,000th birth, but it was still individual and important and deserved to be treated as such. At one point, about an hour after Gabe was born, I was confronted by a nurse, and then more boldly by the head nurse. The argument had to do with an ointment they wanted to put on his eyes.

The ointment contains an antibiotic medication that is designed as a safeguard from unknown, but potential, gonorrheal infection that could have been picked up in the birth canal. Standard medical procedure is a shot of vitamin

K and antibiotic eye ointment given to the baby. I was literally threatened by the head nurse that if I did not allow the application of this ointment on Gabe's eyes, then we would not be allowed to take him home. As I think back, I wonder where he would have lived at the hospital if we were forced to leave without him...

The next day, while Nikki was enjoying some time alone with him, one of the nurses came in and lambasted her for being such a terrible mom for preventing common modalities for her son. This was about the most hurtful thing anyone could have said to a first-time new mother already dealing with the natural effects of the post-birthing process. Needless to say, we saw enough to know future births would be different.

We chose homebirth for our second child, Farrell. She was born in Gabe's room on his bed. It worked well because the twin bed allowed for us to be around Nikki and have easy access to assist her. We had two wonderful midwives and our doula present at the birth. Being at home was accommodating to Nikki's wishes to walk, change positions, and soak in the bathtub, all of which eased labor pain.

Farrell was born without the amniotic sac breaking. This is technically called being "born in the caul." It is a very rare and healthy way of being born, because clearly the baby is protected during the entire birth process. It is odd to see a baby come out within the amniotic sac, however. It is also surprising how strong this sac is. We obviously did get her out of the sac and found out we had a beautiful little girl!

Interestingly enough, there is a medieval myth that babies who are born in the caul are free from the fear of ever dying by drowning. These babies could even sell this caul of protection to others (mainly sailors), as it was highly sought after according to legend. I anecdotally mention this because when Farrell was two, we were at a lodge near the border of Washington and Oregon. They happen to have an Olympic-sized pool, which our family enjoyed by ourselves. Jake was just a baby, so he stayed safely in his carrier. Both Gabe and

Farrell needed our help to get around the pool because even the shallow end was too deep for them. Farrell got tired of this after a while and wanted out. In and out they both went, as it is with kids. They would run over and stick their feet in the hot tub, and then come running back. On one of these trips, Nikki and I were far from where they were jumping in. Farrell thought she had suddenly gained dominance over the water and jumped right in without either of us seeing her. I certainly never swam so fast and will never forget watching her flounder in and out of the water as I struggled to get to her. When I did get to her she was still bobbing for air and may swallowed some water, but was okay and glad to be out of the pool.

Yet that wasn't her only near-escape from drowning. When she was four we were visiting eastern Washington for a go-kart race Gabe was in. The hotel we stayed in had a very small pool. I would estimate it was only fifteen feet by thirty feet. One evening, after a day at the racetrack, the pool area was packed and there must have been over twenty kids in the pool. I was in and out with Farrell, and with a push she was able to swim to the edge on her own from the center. At some point when Nikki and I were out of the pool, Farrell must have jumped into the center from the other side. I don't know how long it was before I noticed her, but once again I was on a rescue mission to save her! When I got her out her lips were slightly blue which was a little scary for all of us.

So much for the legend of the caul. Or, wait—maybe it is working! Now a bit older, she is a fish in the pool.

Within an hour after Farrell was born, the house was cleaned up and cleared out, and we were sitting, holding our new little baby girl. What a precious and special day.

Jake was also born at home. For him, we thought it would be interesting to attempt a water birth, so we planned for and rented a birthing tub and set it up in our living room. Nikki still has a thorn in her side about the fact that at some point she looked up and saw me "working" on my laptop while she was doing her thing in the pool. Truth be told (but she won't listen), I was searching for a web-based timer with a big graphic we could use. I did eventually find one (we are talking about three to five minutes of searching here, okay…), and was able to turn my laptop screen towards us so we could see the exact time Jake was born. Whew! I'm glad I finally got to air the truth around that.

Her labor with Jake was similar to her labor with Farrell, and even shorter in length. We used all of the same methods and included the birthing tub. The part we didn't know about was that it is actually better if I would have gotten in the tub with her and allowed her to sit on my thighs, creating a little canal between my legs for Jake to enter through. As an engineer (and after the fact of course), I have thought many times that a simple seat mechanism would be easy to design for this purpose although I would have been happy to get in with her. Anyway, you can probably guess that she had an extremely bruised and sore tailbone, which made the next few days the most uncomfortable of days after any of the births.

Jake was also nearly born in the caul, which by now we saw as a sign of good health. When his head crowned just seconds before he popped out, the sac broke all in one smooth motion. It was really neat to see all of this and how the water washed him up before he came out for his first breath. Within an hour after he was born, we were once again back to a peaceful home. Nikki rested for a couple hours, because of the soreness of her bum, but was up and about without hesitation soon after.

Summary: Raising Healthy Kids

Raising healthy kids in an unhealthy, toxic world is quite a challenge. There is no perfection. This fact is an important reminder for me because I lean toward idealism in everything. Our kids will be nine, eleven and thirteen this coming summer. We are learning as we go for sure. As we continue to improve and make changes in our choices and understanding, we implement new things for the family as a whole. The kids are quite literally learning with us. Our hope is that we give them the best opportunity possible to avoid many of the bad habits we picked up in our early years. In so doing, the unnatural within our culture will be natural for them and vice versa.

When they were babies, they had breast milk for about eighteen months each. As babies, they also got green barley powder on the pacifier until they were old enough to eat it dry off a spoon. If breast milk is not available, then one recommendation we read was to use 1/3 equal amounts of the following: carrot juice, fresh organic goat's milk, and purified water.

Beyond that, and to keep this pretty simple, we basically just allowed their mouth maturity to determine what they were ready to eat. At a few months, they did not have teeth but were able to use their gums to mash soft fruit. As their teeth came in, they could eat increasingly firmer foods. The infant digestive system development theory is that the digestive system develops at the same rate as the mouth and teeth. In other words, it may not be good to grind up a hard vegetable before they have teeth because the rest of their digestive system may not be ready to handle this sort of food.

Today, the kids generally eat about the same as Nikki and I do. They, like all of us, vacillate between favorite foods. However, the choices they have are always wide open in terms of the vast and broad overall healthy options for nourishment we have available to us. The quantities of food are somewhat self-determined but the items are the same for all.

CHAPTER TWENTY FOUR

Releasing Your Food Chains

It pains me to think of the thousands of people who walk out of doctors' offices and clinics each day, devoid of hope because of their circumstances and what standard protocol has to offer. It breaks my heart to know there are young mothers diagnosed with breast cancer who are being forced to consider the options for their soon-to-be widowed partners and beautiful children. It is a sad picture, but unfortunately these stories and more like this are being played out every day.

Education can come in the form of several options. We can take classes at the local community college, enroll in online curriculums, watch videos, or visit our local library and bookstore. I personally find great solace in the rich mahogany wood of the library, with the tall shelves, comfortable chairs, and spines of educational opportunities displayed before me.

How do you sift through the hundreds of books in the health section of the library or bookstore? To guide your enlightenment in this area. I have provided a list of recommended reading and educational materials in this book. Once you get a taste of what I'm going to share, I hope you'll want to dig in and learn more. There is a sea of misinformation out there and it's important that you have a solid foundation of knowledge upon which to make future decisions. For example, people who are counterfeiters are experts at identifying illegally-produced money. They can spot counterfeit money because they spend an inordinate amount of time studying the real thing. Once they know the real deal like the back of their hand, they can spot a counterfeit quickly and easily. After working through this material, you'll be able to determine truth from fiction on your own.

During my visits to bookstores I often get a spike of excitement when I see a new cover, name, face, or author. The problem for many of us is that we don't know what the motivation is for all these publications. Sadly, most are not as scientific or noble as they lure us to believe. Today, I can flip through these books and quickly determine if they're based on any truth or if they're just more of the same rhetoric that clutters our culture, billboards, advertisements, and our minds. If you first work through some of the resources I list in the recommended resources chapter then you will be armed with the basic knowledge you need to be able to quickly and easily scan these resources and become proficient at determining fact or fiction.

I have covered a variety of topics for you to reference and use this book to guide you through your own journey to your best health. None of the subjects I cover in this book are exhaustive, so I've provided a variety of recommended references and resources where you can dive deeper into the topics that are of greater interest to you. Although I am a huge fan of ongoing reading and education of all kinds, I don't believe you need to spend ten years learning as I have.

I would like you to let me help you over that educational hump and share with you what I've learned. You can use what you glean from my experiences, as well as what you get from other sources, to tailor-make a program that meets your needs and brings you optimal results.

Don't rely just on what other people tell you, however. You need to test things out for yourself. You live in the greatest laboratory you could ever ask for—your own body! A good friend and health advocate references his "brain meter" and his body as a "laboratory of one." This does not mean there is a totally different solution for everyone, similar to what certain diets would espouse. What it does mean is that we are all in different places with differing needs, and we must work with ourselves to grow to a healthy, vibrant existence.

You will need to make some serious decisions about who and what to trust. Our culture will point you to a standard medical doctor (allopathic practitioners) and although they have their place, they are not the supreme experts many would have you believe. In other words, they only know what they know. Like many of us, they've learned from their high school or college teachers and professors, books they've read, and experiences they have been through. Part of their problem is that practicing medicine is their means of survival—that is, how they feed their families, live their dreams, and so on. These doctors are not presented with many opportunities to get first-hand experience with using non-allopathic approaches to physical problems. In my recommendations, I introduce you to some doctors who have traversed this rough road of opposing the standard protocol.

As you continue through the educational process of learning the truth about your health, the full impact of your diet and lifestyle choices on your physical, spiritual, and mental health will become increasingly apparent. This process will force you to reconsider many of the habits and traits that you have picked up through your life from family, friends, or other circumstances where you invested a portion of yourself. I hope that as you do this you will see the necessary changes you need to make are like a child learning to walk. You start with a step, walk a few feet of steps, yards of steps, and then a mile of steps—taking pleasure in the results as you journey.

It is however easier the first time we learn because we do not yet have the food chains strapped on from our previous beliefs. In truth, our parents issue us a set of food chains. Even Nikki and I have done that with our kids because we are still fallible and do not yet know everything there is to know about this topic. Because we started with our own set of food chains, we are still working to break the paradigms that are holding some of those chains in place. The difficulty is never simply learning the steps or understanding the truth. The difficulty is always in getting through your own presuppositions to achieve a new level of understanding. Once you achieve that then change happens effortlessly.

To highlight this, let me share a recent example. We were enjoying a nice lunch at a local salad bar with our kids. Someone who knows our story saw us eating at this particular restaurant and came in. This man's wife is suffering from a number of physical ailments including, but not limited to: cancer, weight control, and mental instability. Her illnesses were warping her entire perspective and their marriage was being threatened by the weight of the physical and spiritual battles being waged. After some greetings at the table, I stepped away with him to talk. His features were set as he flatly stated, "This lifestyle change simply isn't going to work for us—it is simply too difficult and my wife is just not interested." This was shocking to hear. I understand more fully now the ramifications of such a decision.

What many of us suffer from is being stuck in our food chains, which are caused by what we believe and refuse to reconsider.

The changes that I, and many others, suggest are not hard and fast rules. It's not as simple as comparing it to driving north instead of south, using a red pen instead of a black one, or living on the East Coast instead of the West Coast. That's just not the way it is.

We need to be careful to avoid looking at changes or variations in our diet or lifestyle as an all-or-nothing thing. It is a journey, a stairway without an end. It is much like a dimmer switch that controls some lights. A little turn and the lights come on. A bit more turning and the lights get brighter. A standard light switch simply turns the lights on and off all at once. It is, unfortunately, the way many people see their lifestyle choices when in fact we live in a variable world. Our world requires us to consider each of our choices moment by moment.

The big challenge with the all-or-nothing perspective is that it is totally false and even prideful at its core. If you view diet and lifestyle as an all-or-nothing choice then you will never successfully allow yourself to make incremental changes or improvements. You are saying that you need to be perfect or you will not participate. There is folly in the search for perfection. I'm an idealist, so trust me—I deal with this in myself all the time. The truth is that I don't have even a remote chance of achieving perfection. This is difficult for me, and for those around me, because I find it challenging to be satisfied with less than perfection. We will not start if we must start at perfection.

Let me encourage you to ask yourself what incremental changes can be made right now. You may only be able to grasp a very small percentage of the big changes that eventually need to happen. It may seem that the changes you do make feel bigger than they actually are. I remember, during the first few weeks, feeling like I was having my world turned upside down. It felt like I was climbing a huge mountain. Later, as I continued to learn more, I realized that the changes weren't nearly as big of an obstacle as I first imagined them to be. As I got wiser in my understanding, the choices got easier. I could actually recognize where I had more opportunity for improvement, and to this day I am anxious to dive into that.

We need to take steps in the right direction today, more tomorrow, and more each day afterward. The degree of success we have in mastering the choices that impact our daily, physical lives will be in direct relation to our quality and length of life. We may feel we're only achieving slight improvements if we measure our results against a perfect standard, but nothing we ever do will circumvent our need for that standard and, more importantly, our submission to that standard.

Remember, it's a climb. Climbing is challenging, but good in many ways. And, you are never alone!

Closing thoughts

Accept the fact that this is not just about the way you look or feel physically. This is as much a spiritual, emotional, and mental battle as it is a physical one. I can promise you my life has improved immeasurably because of my clarity of mind and loss of fatigue. I think well, I feel better, and I relate in a healthier way. Every aspect of my life is so much better! I know I am a better husband and daddy because I can really think through my relationship with my family as we do life together in good and in challenging times. I believe our lifestyle choices impact our joy. When our minds are clear we can seek and know ourselves and our purpose in a way that simply is not possible within the cloud our culture would have us live within.

CHAPTER TWENTY FIVE

Recommended Resources
Books, Recipes, Videos & Web Sites

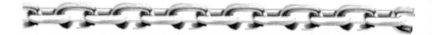

Today we're blessed to have a wealth of information available to us, literally at our fingertips. I believe that you don't have to necessarily agree with, advocate or endorse everything in a book to glean some knowledge from it. The books I recommend are those that I found to be the most truthful. However, even books that don't appear on this list can have nuggets of useful information.

For example, I read *Brain Rules* by John Medina and learned a lot from it. Nevertheless, it was sort of like visiting the National Natural History Museum in Washington, DC, where they call all sorts of animals "family" with the clear and bold intent to teach us through conjecture that man came from animals by evolution. The first chapter of *Brain Rules* covered the effect of exercise on the function of the brain. It is the most comprehensive explanation on the relationship between exercise and brain function I have ever read. Even the author, however, stated that the text, and even all the science combined today, only scratches the surface. He said that at best we should assume what we know is only a very small, nearly immeasurable bit, and that we tend to look at facts and knowledge singularly instead of dynamically amongst the others axioms acting in a particular situation.

While I found *Brain Rules* interesting, I could not help but be a bit distracted and question the foundation of all the information simply due to the pervasive evolutionary theological bent. My point here is that I was able to read the book, and learn from it, even though I knew going in that it was foundationally flawed *(in my view)*. It is nearly impossible to read anything that does not contain at least a bit of untruth, even if it is not intended to be so by the author, publisher, or editors.

Before you dive into the list and make plans for what you will do next, I want to warn you of one other thing that has the ability to hinder us in our path forward. In fact, this little thing can cause us to slip, falter, fall, or worse—to be infected by apathy.

Most of us idolize comfort. We desire to have things done for us, and we work momentarily in anticipation of the promised coming comfort. It could be a meal, a movie with the family, a vacation, or any number of other things. It is clear that we desire comfort over discomfort. When given the choice, the answer is not even a consideration. The reality is that growth always requires pain. There is nothing you have ever learned through education, experience, or revelation that was not delivered on some painful path.

What if I had asked the doctor who removed the mole from my back to have it checked for cancer if he could use something not as sharp, scary, or seemingly painful as the scalpel? What could I suggest that should be used instead? How about a magic wand? In part of my mind, I want to avoid all discomfort at all costs. In the logical part of my mind, I understand that I must endure some pain in order to progress.

We can easily deceive ourselves by creating excuses in our minds for why certain things are okay. For example, I have been told many times by someone that they are following the "blood-type diet" so they can eat _____. Or another one is that this particular thing _____ isn't really that harmful in their view, so they are going to keep doing this and just modify the foundational truths they read. Each of these is like a major blind spot in our minds. It prevents us from seeing the truth that is right in front of us. It quite literally is a link in the chain of our own personal food chains. We press on while dragging carnage from our choices along with us when freedom is quite literally as simple as letting go of the false truths that we keep choosing.

For these reasons, I provide a list of educational recommendations in this section. If you work through these teachings, then you will be armed with the knowledge to be able to determine truth and error.

While I have arranged the books on this list in the order they should be read by people who are just beginning down this path, I would also suggest reading each of these regardless of your place, or the amount of time you have been attempting to live a healthy lifestyle. The one exception is Dr. Russell L. Blaylock's *Natural Strategies for Cancer Patients*. Although this is a great book and filled with great information, it is highly technical, and it is of the most use primarily for allopathic practitioners and people struggling with cancer.

I have also included a list of recipe books we use. This list is simply a sample of the hundred or so recipe books we have collected over the years.

All of these publications should be available at your local library. Or, if your budget and space allows, I recommend purchasing and keeping copies of these on hand for reference and review.

The China Study by T. Colin Campbell

If you like "the data" as much as I do, and you appreciate factual information collected from a reasonable sample size and presented in a simple format, you will enjoy The China Study. I have been told that the source of this data is the largest human study undertaken to prove the relationship between our diet and disease.

Eat to Live by Dr. Joel Fuhrman

What's wrong with the food pyramid, calorie counting, fats, and fish oils? What is this about the calorie-counting myth? Do we really need to eat that much? This book is one of my favorite references for my own education and for assisting others. For example, I love to reference the "Health = Nutrients / Calories" equation, the ideal weight chart, and nutrient density chart. Dr. Fuhrman has an active practice with thousands of patients, and within the hardback edition of this book he shares his findings from years of research, trial, and error.

The Hallelujah Diet by Rev. George Malkmus, Lit.D. with Peter & Stowe Shockey

This is a heartfelt, interesting, story-like publication that demonstrates the overall raw vegan health message. It is as good as any other publication I know of and uses facts, testimonies, stories, results, history, and a Biblical foundation. Our story happens to be included in the cancer section of this publication. The inclusion of our story does not elevate this text on my list. This is a very comprehensive book which combines science, results, and strategies, and can serve as a great handbook for major change in your health. The Hallelujah Diet replaces a previously written and wonderful book titled God's Way to Ultimate Health. I would still strongly recommend this edition because it is more comprehensive and includes a lot of valuable supplemental information.

Excitotoxins by Dr. Russell L. Blaylock

Read what the food manufacturers are adding to the products to entice us to eat them often and in large quantities. Arm yourself with information that will enable you to make sense of at least some of the confusing food labeling. I am convinced that excitotoxins are directly related to the increase in diseases such as Alzheimer's and Lou Gehrig's disease among others.

Natural Strategies For Cancer Patients by Dr. Russell L. Blaylock

Dr. Blaylock talks through the synergistic potential of using natural approaches to fight cancer alongside the conventional medical treatments. Natural Strategies for Cancer Patients is an enjoyable read. It explains the impact and necessity of nutrition in the fight for success over cancer in a scientific (and extremely technical) way that I have not seen in any other book. Dr. Blaylock clearly wrote this text with the intention of bridging the gap between non-allopathic and allopathic approaches. Dr. Blaylock also wrote Excitotoxins, which is in my top five must-reads for anyone truly interested in improving their health.

Roger's Recovery from AIDS by Bob Owen, Ph.D.

I have a special affection for this book because I am the type of person who often finds myself doing what others say is impossible. The book is a true story, and it is as much a love story between old friends as it is a story of the process two men took to prove that AIDS is a lifestyle disease and does not have to be either irreversible or a terminal ailment. I read this book in three hours. Once I started it, I simply could not put it down.

Fast Food Nation by Eric Schlosser

The title of this book is a bit deceiving, but it is nevertheless a worthwhile read. For me it highlighted the industry momentum caused by our cultural choices. These highly-utilized food ingredients are responsible for sicknesses have made it nearly impossible to eradicate illness. Learn how our food industry is controlling our economy, legislation, and most discouraging of all, using up people (mainly migrant workers) as if they were mechanical machines that can be thrown away for a newer version.

Pregnancy, Children, and The Hallelujah Diet by **Olin Idol, N.D., C.N.C**

Dr. Olin Idol does a wonderful job of dispelling many myths in this book. He reviews the basics of such things as natural birthing options, breastfeeding, toxicity, supplements, and more. He also includes instructions on how to transition your child from breast milk to solid foods, and at what age and period of development to consider such changes. We especially appreciate this work because we talk to so many families who say their children simply won't eat a healthy diet. We know, through experience, that children will not starve themselves by refusing to eat healthy food when no unhealthy options are available. This book helps give direction to train your children to eat healthfully and to dispel the misguided training that you may have received as a child.

Raw Knowledge: Enhance the Powers of Your Mind, Body and Soul by **Paul Nison**

Paul interviews a variety of people who have implemented a primarily, or all, raw food diet. Paul is a Hallelujah Acres Health Minister and travels full time speaking and teaching about living a healthy lifestyle. He includes the wisdom of Ana Wigmore and Dr. William Howard Hay, two pioneers in the area of raw, whole, living foods, and discusses the advantages of eating this way for nourishing the human body.

Living Food Cures: The Amazing Stories of 11 People Who Beat Disease Using Raw & Whole Foods by **Joseph R. Farinaccio**

This is an interesting read and contains stories from several people I know. You will be motivated and inspired by these stories. I encourage you to contact these people and bless them if their stories helped you. Most of them have contact information in the book.

Health Via Food by **William Howard Hay, M.D.**

Dr. Hay was a pioneer in true health eighty years ago. He wrote this book in only three weeks in the early 1900's after spending over twenty years attempting to successfully apply the allopathic (modern conventional) approach to medicine. He then spent over twenty years applying natural, diet, and lifestyle-based remedies similar to what we know today with great success. Although he didn't know about the harm caused by animal protein, he was bold enough to face down the status quo and the ridicule of the allopathic practitioners who disagreed with his unconventional approach. Because this book is no longer in print, I found a used, original copy on eBay.

Terapia Gerson Cura Del Cancer Y Otras Enfermedades Cronicas by **Alan Furmanski**

Alan is a melanoma survivor and a health advocate primarily in Spanish-speaking cultures. He introduced himself to me through a mutual friend, and we built a relationship through the years as we both fought to beat the worst, fastest moving cancer. I am very proud of Alan and the work that he continues to do. Since I am not fluent in Spanish, I have not read this book, but Alan has told me that the foundation of it is in and around the teachings of the Gerson Institute.

No More Bull!: The Mad Cowboy Targets America's Worst Enemy: Our Diet by **Howard F. Lyman with Glen Merzer and Joanna Samorow-Merzer**

Howard Lyman is famous for his comments on Oprah regarding the consumption of beef, which lead Oprah to say she would never eat another burger again (because of Mad Cow disease). These comments led to a lawsuit that they won despite the powerful food industry lawyers. Howard grew up on a ranch in Montana, and shares about his experiences in raising cattle and farming. It is interesting to learn about the transition from sustenance farming to production farming or ranching. The farms of today are huge food manufacturing facilities where the ground is the work surface; the seeds, rain, and chemicals are the additives; and the grain or produce becomes the packaged product.

RECIPE BOOKS:

Below is a list of a few of the recipe books we selected from our own collection of over 100 that we own. We generally categorize all of them by recipe difficulty and time to prepare. Many are simple, some fall in the middle, and only a few are really challenging. I have given you a mix of all in order of priority as used or liked in our home. Enjoy!

The favorite recipe book in our home!

Raw Food, Real World by Matthew Kenney & Sarma Melngailis.

We have really enjoyed every single recipe we have ventured into from this book. The raw lasagna is my overall favorite raw food dish. However, the recipes in this book can be moderately difficult to prepare. However, they do a great job of laying out all the ingredients and the tools for the kitchen in this book. It's a must-have piece for any healthy kitchen. And be sure to read the opening pages!

We also enjoy using recipe books by Rhonda Malkmus and Julie Wandling. I especially like Julie's books because they are full of really simple recipes that anyone can make. Julie is a mother of two growing boys and her books are very personal. They tell about her story and are inspiring kitchens across the land. Look for the following titles, _Thank God for Raw_, _Healthy 4 Him_, and _Hallelujah Kids_.

Rhonda's primary book, _Recipes for Life_ is wonderful. It reminds me a bit of the Betty Crocker cookbooks from when I was growing up in the kitchen with my mom. We've had great results and it's not too technical. Be sure to note the 5-star rating system used in this book because it does a great job of helping to educate what foods and combinations are the best for our bodies. Try to lean on the 5-star recipes for staples and splurge with the recipes of lower stars occasionally. The Hallelujah Acres Colonial Bread is amazing. Rhonda also has a really great holiday recipe book that we have used many times. This book is titled *Hallelujah Holiday Recipe Book*.

Vice Cream by Jeff Rogers

Vice Cream should be on the recipe shelf of every vegan. It is packed full of seventy dairy-free frozen dessert recipes. About half of them are raw, but I can promise you all that I have tried are wonderful. Just because you are vegan and eating healthy doesn't mean you can't have ice cream. *My favorite is the basic vanilla!*

Living On Live Food by Alissa Cohen

This is another wonderful recipe book we have added to our library recently. We have made several of the recipes and enjoyed the results.

Raw: The UNcook Book: New Vegetarian Food For Life by Juliano with Erika Lenkert

I met Juliano in his San Monica restaurant. In just a few minutes with him I could tell he was quite the character. Nevertheless, he makes great recipes that result in cuisine-like meals. Just be ready for some hours in the kitchen before you crack this one. The recipes are challenging and include many uncommon ingredients. If you do get it, try the juice called "blood"—it is wonderful.

Juicing For Life: A Guide to the Health Benefits of Fresh Fruit and Vegetable Juicing by Cherie Calbom and Maureen Keane

This is a really useful digest, not only for great juice recipes but also for disease-related information. The recipes in this book are categorized by treatment for certain ailments.

How We All Went Raw: Raw Food Recipe Book by Charles Nungesser and Stephen Malachi

This is a really fun book with many simple recipes that result in some tantalizing meals.

FAVORITE RECIPES:

Visit this page for a bunch of our **favorite recipes**:

This is a wonderful resource because we have loaded many of our favorite recipes for sharing. There's not enough room here to put all of our recipes so we started the online collection and continually add new favorites!

We are also considering doing some food preparation videos so watch for announcements about that.

Basic Salad:

Of course, this isn't the only thing we eat, but getting hooked on good salads is one of the best things that will happen when you begin to make changes in your diet and lifestyle. I estimate that I have had more than 10,000 salads over the last fifteen years, and never once have I eaten the same salad twice. Talk about variety!

Rule number one: Enjoy it! If not, then change it!

We choose to always use 100 percent organic ingredients. The flavor spectrum on conventional produce is the chief reason why people salt their tomatoes and avocados. It is because they don't have any flavor! Eat organic!

Lettuce: Favorites - Butterleaf (nice, thick, and leathery). Sometimes, you might skip the lettuce and have a 'no-lettuce salad.' I also really enjoy hardy romaine leaves for salad or for wraps of all sorts and types. Using the lettuce for the wraps means I do not have to consume a really heavy tortilla.

Tomatoes: Favorites – Heirloom varieties are the best by far, but cherry tomatoes and a few other varieties are also great.

Cucumbers: Remember, there are 170 different ways to slice, cut, chop, etc. Sometimes peel, sometimes not...

Onions: I enjoy green onions or slices of red onion. Be careful with onions. One can be mild while the one next to it can be crazy spicy.

Carrots: We don't use these often in salad, but there are a ton of fun things you can do with them in terms of shape, etc. I recently got some fun peelers that enable the carrots to be pealed with fun grooves and used as is or they can then be sliced which really shows off their neat shapes.

Avocado: They need to be pretty firm or they are gross, but if they are ripe, they are amazing. You can also make a guacamole and top the salad with it and some salsa.

Spices: Sometimes I just go in and begin dumping various spices, but one that sticks in my mind is fennel seed. It is nice if it gets a chance to soak it in, for instance, some rice wine vinegar or some other liquid in the bottom of your salad to bring out the flavor.

Sauces/dressings: Go wild here, but remember that the more exotic you get with your sauce, the fewer ingredients you need to be really satisfying. You can kill the value of some ingredients by over-dressing. I love just freshly squeezed lemon—and depending upon the salad—no dressing at all can be nice.

Toppings: We have a cupboard full of nuts, seeds, raisins, flax, etc. I may take chopped walnuts with oranges on one salad, with cashews or sunflower seeds on another salad, or a combination of any of these. We also really enjoy a raw taco mix made mainly from walnuts. Topping your salad with it makes it a taco salad!

Shocking: For fun, try blending your salad sometime. You can easily get hooked on these...

ENJOY! And remember to visit www.freggies.com regularly to see our favorite recipes.

AUDIO/VIDEO RESOURCES:

Forks Over Knives by friends Dr. T. Colin Campbell and Dr. Caldwell Esselstyn. This film is an enjoyable and educational documentary done primarily by two doctors who do not need to produce such a piece but wanted to in an effort to further the information they have learned over 40+ years of study and experience. We took our kids to a pre-screening of this movie in a theater and really enjoyed it.

Fat, Sick & Nearly Dead by Joe Cross is a really fun documentary film explaining the life of Joe as he struggled with his own food chains. After years of bobbing up and down on the scale, the Aussie decided to come to America— but with a twist; he was not going to eat our food! He spent a month in New York drinking only his own fresh juices. It was a good place to start as there are a lot of wonderful juice bars in New York. He spent another month driving across America. He met some amazing people along the way, heard their stories, and lost a lot of weight. Joe mentioned to me recently that he is working on another film as well, so watch for that to be released.

The Miraculous Self-Healing Body by Hallelujah Acres, includes professional insight on the subject of and relationship between diet and disease from four medical doctors, doctors Neal Barnard, M.D.; John McDougall, M.D.; Joel Fuhrman, M.D.; and Russell Blaylock, M.D. This video, narrated by Rev. George Malkmus, Lit.D., is part of the Hallelujah way of teaching and the truth in the message is powerful and inspiring. I think our culture's respect for doctors is part of what makes this particular educational piece carry such impact.

Super-Size Me was released in 2005, and is a story of a guy who eats only McDonald's food for thirty days and filmed his entire experiment. It was really an interesting and worthwhile investment of a couple of hours. It helped me come up with my perspective on food production in our culture today. It goes like this (in my mind at least): there are basically two rules that matter in food production in our culture. The first rule is that the food cannot cause immediate death to the customer. That's right, you may die from eating it over and over, but that seems to be okay in our society. It may be loaded with MSG, and you may feel terrible, but as long as your taste buds are tantalized, the food will sell. After all, if there are side effects to the food we eat, there most certainly must be a pill we can take to curb the side effects (I won't go on about the profit machines called pharmaceutical companies and how a drug has never cured anything...). The second rule is that the food has to be profitable. These companies are in business. Food manufacturing is about money. This is not a healthy vs. non-healthy issue. Even the farms are making money! These are just the facts, and it is our responsibility to be aware of them. Food is a very big business and the results of the profit machines are not always healthy for us. (Available in DVD format from any public video rental location and may be found in some health food stores).

Food, Inc. was released in theaters June of 2009. It is the highest quality and most comprehensive movie I've seen showing the relationship between our consumer purchases and the products of the food industry. It is argued that the food industry is leading the population astray with unhealthy, yet profitable, foods (what they call food), though they would defend themselves by saying they are simply producing the things people want to buy. Learn more at www.foodincmovie.com.

Fast Food Nation started as a book by Eric Schlosser, but was later made into a B- grade movie with a cameo by Bruce Willis, where he tags the famous American meal as the '$*!# burger.' I think the tag-line they have for the movie is great, "Would you like lies with that?" By the name, you would believe this film has a lot to do with fast food or fast food restaurants. In reality, it has more to do with the sad story of the mechanism or machine that quite literally uses up and eats humans in the process—namely and chiefly U.S. migrants from Mexico. If you can watch the last ten minutes of the movie, and still stomach lunch that includes some form of animal products, then you have scales of steel and calluses that need a grinder.

God's Way To Ultimate Health by Hallelujah Acres, starring Rev. George Malkmus, is the video our family watched that blustery, but insightful, Christmas day of 1999. It is basically an overview of what the whole Hallelujah Diet® and Lifestyle message is about. It has been updated since and is even better now. The information is irrefutable and has universal application to all people. If you are starting down this path, I would suggest getting a copy for your library and schedule a couple hours to watch it about every three to six months during the first two years of treatment. I am still amazed how much I learn as I watch it fifty times over.

Eating by Mike Anderson is a very informative video that uncovers many facts the meat and dairy industries don't want you to know, mainly that the products of these industries are the biggest cause of disease and death in the western culture. Anderson discusses the link between diet and disease in America. His presentation is a bit disturbing but his heart is to expose how our farms have turned into factories whose chief purpose is feeding the animals we eat.

Apps & Web Destinations:

VegOut
Great app we have used many times when traveling to find a place close to wherever we are that serves healthy options.

MealLogger
Good app to track and get social around your food.

Hope4Health.org
You may have already visited, but this is our little website. It has a number of resources but one that is really interesting if the PerforMAX Challenge where you can assess your overall healthfulness currently. Check it out!

Hacres.com
This is Hallelujah Acres main website. There are tons of testimonies, resources and products! Tell them that Jerrod and Nikki Sessler sent you if you call. Many of the staff there know us and they will likely give you a discount!

Good 2 Go Café
We have a vision to place healthy cafés across the country in strategic community locations. These cafés will be owned

and staffed by people with a passion for teaching and assisting people in eating healthy food, as well as learning more about the food they eat and how the lifestyle they live impacts their overall health. Part of the café concept is that we will also deliver fresh, organic produce regionally in and around the café through Freggies. So, check out www.freggies.com and tell us if you are interested in starting a produce delivery service or launching a healthy café in your region.

HACO TACO (hacotaco.com)

We have long visited restaurant after restaurant in search of the perfect place to eat that is fresh, fun, healthy, and where we can eat anything on the menu any time of day any day of the week. Even though we own the brand, we do not eat there every day but it sure is nice to have a place to go when we want. HACO TACO is a franchise concept so we are expanding it to other towns, cities, states and even other countries! Our family is learning Spanish so we spent some time in Central America where they love tropical produce, fresh food and tacos—fish tacos to be specific! We were hooked and the vision for HACO TACO came to life.

Freggies.com

An organic produce delivery services Nikki and I started to meet the needs of busy families who wanted access to great quality organics at a bit lower price than retail, on their terms (pick what you want), with free delivery! We are now expanding Freggies into other cities, which opens up franchise opportunities for people in other cities. Note: Make sure to pronounce "Freggies" correctly... It sounds like "veggies." Just drop the "V" and add an "Fr" from "Fruit" or "Fresh". Fresh Fruit & Veggies = Freggies! Yes, we know that phonetically, it should have only one 'g,' but it jives better with "Fruit & Veggies" as Freggies!

APPENDIX A

Jerrod Sessler Cancer Diagnosis Timeline:

This section is a reference for those who are really interested in the process we went through and the choices we made. You have to realize we didn't really know much about, nor believe in the idea of the natural self-healing ability of our bodies at the start of this. The education process however grew rapidly as the weeks, months and years clicked by. At a certain point only a few weeks into the learning curve, we got to a point where we trusted what we thought to be true enough to place the balance of my life in the hands of that truth.

12/31/98 First doctor's visit when the mole on my back was discussed. I mentioned the mole on my back that was bothering me with an itching sensation. This doctor looked at it and said it looked fine. He did not document this, but did note discussing my dry skin.

For anyone interested in the resolution to this obvious failure by someone in the medical profession, I want to elaborate a bit here. In other words, did we sue the doctor? The answer is no. There are fundamentally two reasons. The first is that I struggle with the criteria our culture uses when engaging the legal system. I am not saying that there is not just cause for such actions at times, but I don't know if this was one of those. The second, and more resounding, reason is that I believe this was providential by God. Sort of like when he closed Pharaoh's mind to the common sense of letting the Israelite slaves go, even when God's wrath was upon him and his Egyptian people repeatedly. I believe God blocked the doctor from warning me about this mole, possibly along with everyone else, until it was the right time to illuminate the course of action I needed to take. The reason I believe this is primarily because I know myself, and I know I probably would not have taken such serious action had I not been faced with a literal death sentence. Had I thought maybe I had a fifty percent chance of making it, I would have taken it. Thus, I would now be dead because it would not have worked. We know from history that melanoma returns with a vengeance, and the patients are rarely spared when conventional medical treatments are enacted. Now, I get to live a wonderful life with a gorgeous wife, incredible children, and loving family. I get to glorify God and live out His joy for me daily.

10/12/99   I showed my mom (who happens to be a nurse) the mole and said it was itching. She stated she would get me into a dermatologist as soon as possible. I trusted her and agreed. My mom had seen the mole before, but it had been a long time before, and she had chiefly just seen me backing up to wall corners to scratch it.

My weight at this point: 217 (the highest ever....)

10/13/99   Mom went to work the next morning and promptly called to schedule an appointment with Dr. A. However she was booked more than a month out, so Mom asked who could get me in, and Dr. B had an opening on the 19th. Dr. B was a new doctor, so Mom couldn't ask anyone about her. However, Mom went by the clinic reputation of hiring good doctors and she made the appointment, time being of the essence.

10/19/99	I saw Dr. B and she set up an appointment to excise the lesion. She stated that she didn't think it was anything, but it could be a basal cell carcinoma. I told her that my maternal grandfather had a history of melanoma.
10/24/99	I called Mom, wanting to video my excision. She didn't think Dr. B would appreciate that, but told me I could call and ask them.
11/4/99	Doctor's notes: Excision lesion/mole on back (1.5 x 4.0 cm) excision.

I called Mom from Dr. B's waiting area to come down and observe the excision, since we weren't recording it by video. They took me back with Mom while Nikki stayed in the waiting area, and Mom went back also. Dr. B came in and inked the shape and size of her intended incision. Dr. B's assistant numbed the area with a local anesthetic and Dr. B came in, gowned and gloved. She made slow scalpel cuts to excise the mole, which came out in one piece. She also made small scraping and digging type cuts at the body edge of the cut in some areas. Dr. B sewed two layers, pulling my back together fairly firmly. Before the stitching was complete I complained that I was starting to feel it, but I was fine and she was to continue. She and her assistant applied a pressure dressing and told me to keep it on for at least twenty-four hours before removing or showering. During this visit I stated that Mom was to have any reports or access to my records while we were in the room.

The five Clark levels of invasion for melanoma:

Level I: Melanomas confined to the outermost layer of the skin, the epidermis. Also called *melanoma in-situ*.

Level II: Penetration by melanomas into the second layer of the skin, the dermis.

Levels III-IV: Melanomas invade deeper through the dermis, but are still contained completely within the skin.

Level V: Penetration of melanoma into the fat of the skin beneath the dermis, penetration into the third layer of the skin, the subcutis.

11/6/99   I asked Mom if she could take out the stitches, and she said she wouldn't mind at all. I said it would save me a trip downtown. I also asked her to cancel my appointment, which she did the next morning.

11/11/99   *Doctors notes: Dermatopathology Report by Dr. C – Malignant melanoma Clark's Stage IV - Read out as 1.14 mm in depth and within 1mm of the excisional margin.* (see note at the end of the chronology addressing level and stage issues / contradiction)

Mom called to see if the report was in yet, and when she was told that it had not come in, she asked to be called when the pathology report did arrive. The person at the other end of the phone agreed. They did not inform her that Dr. B was out of town, or that Mom could not have the report or that they needed a release.

11/16/99   Biopsy results visit with Dr. B. After initially discounting the severity of the melanoma, Dr. B consulted with Dr. A and decided to send me to the local melanoma clinic. She did a full body skin check for other lesions and reminded me to use sunscreen lotion. She also sent me for a chest x-ray and liver function tests for metastases.

I want to note here that I included the reference from the doctor about using sun screen as a point of clarity. I did have a few sunburns as a child and as I grew up. I grew up primarily in the

Pacific Northwest where short bursts of sun, rather than regular baking, are common. I do not, however, believe that the skin cancer is a direct relationship to sun exposure. Excessive toxins within my body caused the cancer I had during a time when I was nutritionally deficient and could not prevent the creation and spreading of the cancerous cells.

11/16/99 After not hearing for such a long time, Mom called to get the report results. They said that it had gone to Dr. C and gave her the number. She called and they faxed the report right over saying that it had been sent to Dr. B long ago. When she received the fax, she was shocked.

Mom called my sister to see if perhaps Deirdre knew if I had gotten any report. Deirdre called me and I reported that I had not heard a word. I knew that Mom had called her, and I could hear in her voice the news was not good, even though she didn't mention it directly. Then Mom called me and told me to call Dr. B's office and ask for the results. I called Mom back later and said that I was going to pick up Nikki, and would be seeing the doctor at 4:30. I asked her if she would come down.

When I arrived, I called Mom and she came down, meeting a worried Nikki in the hall near the office. We all went in the room together. Dr. B came in and told us the news very calmly as if it was no big deal. She said she would just do a wide excision in the office and that would be that. She measured the width she wanted to make, the wide excision pointing to an area approximately two centimeters from the original incision in all directions. Mom said nothing in this visit except to ask at what point it becomes surgical instead of dermatological. Dr. B answered that usually they (dermatologists) took care of it until it became a skin graft situation. She said she would have to do a full skin check today. At this point, Nikki and Mom started to leave, and I said that since Mom gave birth to me and Nikki sees me everyday, there was no reason for them to leave. Dr. B looked me over and found one other suspicious area on my left buttock that she thought would need to come out. She left the room for a few minutes and then came back and said that she had spoken with Dr. A, and would refer me to the local melanoma clinic for possible lymph mapping. Dr. B seemed to take this quite lightly and stated that where she came from, they didn't consider this level to need lymph mapping and insinuated that it was overkill. She said her assistant would get the number for us. Mom volunteered her extension.

11/17/99 Mom knew someone with the number for the local melanoma clinic, so both Nikki and Mom called. The assistant at the local melanoma clinic was very nice, but said I couldn't get in until the 30th. Mom explained that this had been progressing for a while and that we would be available any time if she could find a cancellation spot. The lady said if Mom could make copies of the records and fax them to her and hand-carry the slides, she could look for another spot. Mom got the chart, made copies and faxed them to her, and in the meantime she reworked her schedule and called us both back to say the new time and date would be 11/23/99 at 10:30.

11/18/99 Mom tried to reach someone at Dr. C's office, but got only voice mail, so she left a message saying she would like to pick up the slides about 12:00 noon. When she arrived at the doctor's office, they were unaware she had been coming because that nurse was off and the voice messages had not been listened to. They did look for them while she sat a bit. Soon they came out saying the slides went back to Dr. B's office as per her protocol. Dr. B's office had not said anything about the local melanoma clinic needing records, or that they had the slides and would be glad to provide them to us.

11/19/99 Mom called and asked to be able to pick up the slides, and Dr. B personally spoke to Mom about the fact that she needed a written release. Mom asked if my statements in our visits were not enough. Dr. B said no. Mom asked if she had to call me off the job to come down and fill out the form. Dr. B said it could be faxed. Mom still had to reach me out on the road to have me go home to get the fax and return it signed, etc. This was the last straw for her. She started to cry and had difficulties the rest of the day. She took a walk at lunchtime and stopped back by Sandra's office in staffing to see if she could get the day off to go with us to the local melanoma clinic. Sandra looked at her and asked what was wrong, and Mom burst into tears. It seemed as if Dr. B and her office staff just didn't care and were more worried about protocol than the patient or patient care and needs. To top it off, they turned Mom in for getting the chart and copying it for Dr. D at the local melanoma clinic. First off, she did nothing until the pathology report was late and no one had called. She followed all the rules to the "T." The fact that there was no cooperation or concern left her feeling that if she requested anything, it would not get done.

A staff member in the human resources department called Mom down to speak to her about ordering a chart, and copying it when it was not her doctor's chart duty. She just explained that she got it for the local melanoma clinic's copies, out of lack of confidence in Dr. B's office. They had not demonstrated any professional courtesy, respect for patient intention, or concern for the other clinic's/patient's "need to know," or the fact that she was the most logical access to any of the above. They didn't care about anything but their rules.

Dr. B's office should have had a policy whereby positive pathology reports were given to another physician to evaluate and arrange to call the patient. They should have offered a release at anytime when we were there together. They should have said that the local melanoma clinic would need records and slides, and they would be glad to help expedite that. They could have offered Mom the slides and asked that she follow up with the signed consent.

My mom is a wonderful sweet woman who has served in the medical community the majority of her life. The depiction above is more of a mother who was worried for her son than who she really is or how she normally acts. I am encouraged and proud of my mom because she has fully adopted a primarily raw, vegan lifestyle and she is much healthier herself than she was at this time. To clarify, at the time, she was working in the medium-sized clinic in Seattle where this all started. My mom also accompanied us to nearly all of our appointments the first few months.

11/23/99 Mom, Nikki, and I had the first appointment with Dr. D, and we all liked him very much. He was quite upbeat and nice. The whole group at the local melanoma clinic treated us with the utmost courtesy and concern. They were totally comfortable with the family visit.

11/23/99 *Doctor's notes: Initial visit schedule with Dr D, local melanoma clinic Surgeon for wide excision and sentinel lymph node mapping of the mole excision area.*

12/2/99 I had the lymph mapping, another mole excised, and the wide excision on my back.

12/14/99 Mom, Nikki, and I went to my appointment to get results and have my stitches removed. The incisions looked fine and Dr. D took the stitches out. The pathology, however, was not good. One node (the sentinel) was positive, and Dr. D would have to do a full excision of the lymph nodes in the left axilla (armpit), which would leave me somewhat concave, permanently numb in some areas, and recuperating for weeks with limited mobility.

12/16/99 *Doctors notes: CT scan to clear the liver of cancer — negative.*

12/21/99 Consultation with oncologist, Dr. E, who suggested Interferon for one year with intravenous injections of 20 million units on Mondays and Fridays, followed by eleven months of 10 million units subcutaneously Mondays, Wednesdays, and Fridays. They also offered a randomized trial study treatment of a new vaccine, Melacine, plus lower doses of Interferon for a total of two years.

Mom, Nikki and I met with Dr. E, the oncologist. He told us that he and Dr. D had reviewed the pathology report, and felt that it should have been a 2.3-millimeter melanoma instead of a 1.14-millimeter, which is a substantial difference. The CT scan was fine. They recommended Interferon treatment, or the randomized study of Interferon, or Interferon and Melacine. He went over all the possible side effects to the drugs, which were two year's worth of the worst fatigue and depression I could ever imagine, as well as possible destruction of other cells and hair loss, and such.

Dr. E informed us of the overall prognosis at this point. He indicated that he believed my chances were about 5 percent chance overall to live ten or more years thus the title of my first book. He also said that I likely had a forty percent chance of a five-year survival rate. If I choose to succumb to the chemical treatments he was recommending, he felt I could improve my odds by fifteen percent overall.

This was also the meeting when Dr. E informed us we would not be able to have children and that my racing career was over. Mom, Nikki, and I would always pray at these meetings, but this was one of the most difficult and, I believe, the only one we cried at. After Dr. E left the room, we huddled together, wept, and prayed.

12/21/99 *Doctors notes: Second opinion of the original dermopathology suggested that it had been read incorrectly and was actually 2.3mm because it had actually followed a hair follicle down.* (see note at the end of the chronology addressing level and stage issues / contradiction)

12/27/99 I had surgery to have my whole auxiliary lymphatic system removed. I had a drain in for a week or so, and waited for the biopsy report until Thursday just before the New Year. Basically what that meant was they cut open my left armpit and cut all the lymph system out. At the time of this operation, I weighed 213 pounds.

OF NOTE: This was just two days after we watched the *How to Eliminate Sickness* video (now called: God's Way to Ultimate Health). I remember lying on the bed waiting to be wheeled into the operation room, thinking to myself, "What on earth am I doing? I know this is wrong, but everyone around me wants me to do it. If I get out of this bed, my family will flip out and everyone will think I am crazy." In retrospect, and especially after going through the weeks that followed this surgery, I wish I had jumped off that bed and walked out of the hospital!

This was really the start of the self-healing journey for us. I just wish I had started just a little bit sooner. The encouragement and support from my family was important during this time, but the pressure to do what the doctors said was overwhelming. Our education did increase, as did our faith, in what we now know to be true.

1/4/00   Appointments to have the drain taken out or checked, and results of the biopsy (which were not available before the holiday).

Doctor's notes: Postoperative visit with Dr. D.

1/11/00   I had an appointment with Dr. F, an oncologist. This appointment with Dr. F was both frustrating and enlightening. We explored the survival rates, actual causes of cancer (per standard medical assumptions) and carcinogen effects, the poor prognosis of recurrence, and the treatment options available. Even then he would not give me more than a sixty percent chance of survival without high-dose Interferon, Melacine, or Interluken. These treatments would raise the survival chance to about seventy to seventy-five percent. He said they had no way to know if there were any more tumors until it could be too late. His advice included, primarily, the high-dose Interferon, and secondarily, the study with Interferon and Melacine. He did not know of another way to get the vaccine other than at the local melanoma clinic. He did not think the consultant that group hired to do the research was of much value, stating that he or we could pull it right off the Internet ourselves. He also believed in vitamin E, Selenium, and vitamin C combined with a healthy diet, but said they did not have data to prove that any diet helped. He said the Interluken, while given only a few months instead of a year or two, was so toxic it had a small chance of killing me while trying to kill the cancer. Dr. F actually got very hostile when I mentioned not taking the standard treatment, and Mom felt really bad because she had recommended Dr. F as a second source.

1/13/00 My initial visit with Dr. G, a naturopath. Dr. G recommended several dietary restrictions and several supplements. I started taking his list of supplements, which was about $600 per month. He also suggested a diet without red meat, dairy, or simple carbohydrates. He also suggested increasing seafood, soy, green tea, fruits, vegetables, legumes, whole grains, yams, squash, olive oil, nuts, and seeds. Dr. G recommended 20mg of melatonin at bedtime to slow growth of abnormal cells. I slowly quit taking all the supplements over a six-month period after starting. They just seemed like a waste of money, and only really applicable for someone who refused to change what they were eating. Since I was fully adopting a healthy diet and lifestyle, I didn't feel like I needed all those supplements.

OF NOTE: I did eat seafood as a transitional food about once a quarter for the first year, but eventually lost the desire for it. That is better because there are some serious mercury issues with seafood. In *Eat to Live*, by Dr. Joel Fuhrman, he identifies which types of seafood are known to be worse than others for the mercury issue. I am not advocating that you eat any seafood, but if you are going to use it as I did once in a while, then you should know as much as you can about it.

4/00   My first three-month visit. "All looks good." I had lost a lot of weight, and they said I was doing really well. "Whatever you are doing, keep it up."

7/00   "Wow," they said, "you have lost over forty pounds, you look great. Seriously, what are you doing? We don't need to see you for another six months."

1/9/01   One year follow-up visit with Dr. D. No evidence of recurrent melanoma. He agreed with our diet and lifestyle approach, but expressed concern that I may not be able to sustain the lifestyle long-term. This proved his wisdom, because we live in an unhealthy culture, but also proved that he didn't know me or the level of desire I have for life and my aspirations. "No need to come in every six months for these visits. See you in a year!" That final visit never did happen.

1/02   Final CAT scan which was, like the rest, clear. Lots of detail is missing in the chronology above. One stark omission is the dates and appointments with another dermatologist who I will refer to as Dr. H once I gather up the info. I saw him in three-month intervals for the first year, and then six months the second year. We did CAT scans every six months, but I need to dig up all the data on that as well.

I lost about forty pounds the first year, and then it seemed to level off for a year or more. Then I lost another twenty pounds, and I have pretty much stayed between 155-165 ever since.

CLARIFICATION:

The survival percentages quoted on 1/11/00 were from a different doctor in a different clinic, and this was the first visit where he had no prior knowledge of my situation. These survival estimates are radically different than the ones given to us by the local melanoma clinic, and I do not know on what they are based. I assume it's a professional guess.

On 1/11/00, the doctor mentions "the fear of returning melanoma," which tends to be even scarier than a first diagnosis because it often returns internally, advances very fast, and attacks critical, high blood-flow organs such as the heart, brain, and lungs. The doctors at the local melanoma clinic corroborated this information.

Throughout the first few years following my diagnosis, there was a lot of confusion on the actual level or stage of my diagnosis. We have documented proof that the various doctors did not agree in the staging, or established the level because of their process of reading the scans of the actual mole. These diagnoses are confused by different measurement types as well. The two types referred to in my story are Staging (stage 1 through 5, where 5 is the worst case), which is commonly used among many cancers, and Clark's Level (Clark's Level 1-5—see chart), which is specific to melanoma cancer. My diagnosis was a Stage 3 and Clark's Level 4, based on the information we have gathered. We were, however, told it was Stage 4 once it was confirmed that it had spread to the lymph system. There was also a discrepancy in the way the depth was measured because it was much deeper along a hair follicle than the rest of the mole. I also find the Clark's Level rather confusing because the cancer had spread, but the definitions for the levels don't specifically cover that type of situation.

OF NOTE: This whole thing makes me wonder what else I don't know. Or another way of putting it is, "What else am I totally clueless about?" This life change was so radical for us that we were profoundly impacted at the core of our belief system. We were not arrogant enough to think we knew it all, but this whole idea that the foods we were eating were actually causing the diseases was astounding. It made us wonder, and possibly opened ourselves up to the Spirit of Truth even more. Hopefully that has enabled us to fully live the lives God intended for us because we are less likely to accept something "just because it has always been that way." I want to challenge you to question what you believe and verify that it is in full alignment with Truth. Thank God we have Truth as a frame of reference for everything in life.

SOURCES

Listed below are the sources from which I took direct quotes, cited specific facts, or was otherwise informed during the writing of this book. Website URLs are current as of January 2014.

About Freggies. (n.d.). *FREGGIES*. Retrieved January 4, 2014, from http://www.freggies.com/coop/

Blaylock, R. L. (19981997). *Excitotoxins the taste that kills*. Santa Fe, N.M.: Health Press.

Blaylock, R. L. (2003). *Natural strategies for cancer patients*. New York: Twin Streams.

Calbom, C., & Keane, M. (1992). *Juicing for life*. Garden City Park, N.Y.: Avery Pub. Group.

Campbell, T. C., & Campbell, T. M. (2005). *The China study: the most comprehensive study of nutrition ever conducted and the startling implications for diet, weight loss and long-term health*. Dallas, Tex.: BenBella Books.

Cohen, A. (20062004). *Living on live food* (4th ed.). Kittery, Me.: Cohen Pub. Co..

Collins, J. C. (2001). *Good to great: why some companies make the leap-- and others don't*. New York, NY: HarperBusiness.

Anderson, M. (Director). (2002). *Eating* [Documentary]. United States of America: Ravediet.com.

(2007). Episode 120 [Television series episode]. In *How It's Made*. Seattle: Discovery Channel.

Linklater, R. (Director). (2007). *Fast food nation* [Documentary]. United States of America: 20th Century Fox Home Entertainment.

Cross, J. (Director). (2011). *Fat, sick & nearly dead* [Documentary]. Australia, USA: Reboot Holdings.

Kenner, R. (Director). (2010). *Food, inc* [Documentary]. United States of America: CTV International [ed.] :.

Fulkerson, L. (Director). (2012). *Forks over knives* [Documentary]. United States of America: Monica Beach Media :.

Francis M. Pottenger, Jr.. (2013, November 30). *Wikipedia*. Retrieved January 5, 2014, from http://en.wikipedia.org/wiki/Francis_M._Pottenger,_Jr.

Fuhrman, J. (2011). *Eat to live: the amazing nutrient-rich program for fast and sustained weight loss* (Rev. ed.). New York: Little,

Brown and Co..

Genetically modified organism. (2014, April 1). *Wikipedia*. Retrieved January 4, 2014, from http://en.wikipedia.org/wiki/Genetically_modified_organism

Gerson, C., & Bishop, B. (2009). (1a ed.). Mexico?: Editorial Alan Furmanski.

Gluttony. (2013, December 27). *Wikipedia*. Retrieved January 7, 2014, from http://en.wikipedia.org/wiki/Gluttony

Malkmus, G. (Director). (0). *God's Way to Ultimate Health* [Documentary]. United States of America: Hallelujah Acres.

Hallelujah Acres. (n.d.). *Vegetarian Recipes, Healthy Eating Hallelujah Diet:*. Retrieved January 5, 2014, from http://www.hacres.com/

Idol, O. (2002). *Pregnancy, children & the Hallelujah diet*. Shelby, NC: Hallelujah Acres Publishing.

Kenney, M., Melngailis, S., & Karetnick, J. (2005). *Raw food, real world: 100 recipes to get the glow*. New York: Regan Books.

Lenkert, E. (1999). *Raw: the uncook book*. New York: Regan Books.

Lewis, C. S. (2001). *The Screwtape letters: with Screwtape proposes a toast*. San Francisco: HarperSanFrancisco.

Lyman, H. F., Merzer, G., & Merzer, J. (2005). *No more bull!: the mad cowboy targets America's worst enemy, our diet*. New York: Scribner.

Malkmus, G. H., Shockey, P., & Shockey, S. (2006). *The Hallelujah diet: experience the optimal health you were meant to have*. Shippensburg, PA: Destiny Image Publishers.

Malkmus, R. J. (2005). *Hallelujah holiday recipes: from God's garden*. Shelby, NC: Hallelujah Acres Pub..

Medina, J. (2008). *Brain rules: 12 principles for surviving and thriving at work, home, and school*. Seattle, WA: Pear Press.

Metastatic Melanoma Survival Story. (n.d.). *Metastatic Melanoma Survival Story*. Retrieved January 7, 2014, from http://www.hope4health.org/

Nungesser, C. J., & Nungesser, G. M. (2004). *How we all went raw*. Mesa, Ariz.: In the Beginning Health Ministry.

Organic food. (2014, March 1). *Wikipedia*. Retrieved January 7, 2014, from http://en.wikipedia.org/wiki/Organic_food

Owen, B. (1987). *Roger's recovery from AIDS*. Malibu, CA: DAVAR.

Rogers, J. (2004). *Vice cream: gourmet vegan desserts*. Berkeley, Calif.: Celestial Arts.

Seuss, D. (1990). *Oh, the places you'll go!*. New York: Random House.

Spurlock, M. (Director). (2004). *Super size me* [Documentary]. United States of America: Warner Home Video.

Surveillance, Epidemiology, and End Results ProgramTurning Cancer Data Into Discovery. (n.d.). *Melanoma of the Skin.* Retrieved January 5, 2014, from http://seer.cancer.gov/statfacts/html/melan.html

The Food Journal ThatTalks Back.. (n.d.). *MealLogger Photo Food Journal.* Retrieved January 7, 2014, from http://www.meallogger.com/

Barnard, N. (Director). (2009). *The Miraculous Self-Healing Body* [Documentary]. United States of America: Hallelujah Acres.

VegOut - Vegetarian Restaurant Guide for the iPhone. (n.d.). *VegOut - Vegetarian Restaurant Guide for the iPhone.* Retrieved January 7, 2014, from http://vegoutapp.com/

Wandling, J. (2002). *Thank God for raw: recipes for health.* Akron, OH.: Healthy 4 Him Pub..

Wandling, J. (2003). *Healthy 4 Him: recipes for healthy living.* Shelby, N.C.: Hallelujah Acres.

Wandling, J. (2005). *Hallelujah kids: resource for moms : recipes for kids.* Shelby, N.C.: Hallelujah Acres.

organic. (n.d.). *Dictionary.com.* Retrieved January 5, 2014, from http://dictionary.reference.com/browse/organic

Jerrod Sessler

After being given a five percent chance of surviving advanced-stage melanoma skin cancer, author, speaker, entrepreneur, and father, Jerrod Sessler decided to take responsibility not only for his recovery but for his health as well. Jerrod's story is a riveting message of hope and healing that will inspire you. His delivery is full of energy and enthusiasm for the health message that has become his passion—a message that he says is very basic but much obscured by our culture. Jerrod speaks regularly on the topics of health, racing, and faith.

Jerrod has earned multiple engineering degrees along with multiple certifications and recognitions from associations such as the *Small Business Administration, Entrepreneur Magazine,* the *International Franchise Association, Hallelujah Acres* and the *National Heritage Foundation.* Jerrod is an honored veteran, serves as a PCO and volunteer lobbyist in Washington State and in Washington, DC, is a successful entrepreneur, and serves in several non-profit foundations. He has also gained recognition as a successful NASCAR Driver.

Contact Jerrod:

Thank you for reading Food Chains. To connect with or follow Jerrod, please leverage one of the following methods:

Google+: https://plus.google.com/+JerrodSessler

Facebook: https://www.facebook.com/jerrod.sessler

Twitter: @Sessler

Web: www.hope4health.org; www.jerrodsessler.com; www.freggies.com; www.hometask.com

Thank you for sharing your ideas to improve the clarity of this book and for noting pesky little errors: feedback@todoblue.com